Natural Treatment Solutions For Hyperthyroidism and Graves' Disease

*Discover How Following A Natural Thyroid
Treatment Protocol Can Restore Your Health...
And Help You To Avoid Radioactive Iodine*

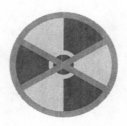

Eric M. Osansky, D.C.

Natural Treatment Solutions for Hyperthyroidism and Graves' Disease
By Eric M. Osansky, DC

Printed in the United States of America

Natural Endocrine Solutions
4100 Carmel Road Ste B #106
Charlotte, NC 28226

www.GravesDiseaseBook.com

Book design: Adina Cucicov, Flamingo Designs

ISBN: 978-0-615-48493-8

A Word Of Caution To The Reader

This book is for informational and educational purposes only, and is not meant to be used as medical advice or as a recommended treatment protocol for people with hyperthyroidism or Graves' Disease. As stated in the book, people with any type of hyperthyroid disorder should not self-treat their condition. The author does not take responsibility for any possible consequences resulting from any person taking action after reading this book. The publication of this book does not act as a replacement for consulting with a competent healthcare professional. Before engaging in any type of treatment, diet, nutritional supplements and/or herbs, exercise, or any other action mentioned in this book, it is highly recommended to consult with your physician, or another competent healthcare professional.

Dedication

I dedicate this book to people with hyperthyroid conditions who are looking to do everything possible to preserve the health of their thyroid gland, and therefore avoid radioactive iodine or thyroid surgery.

Acknowledgements

First of all, I'd like to thank my wonderful wife Cindy for her continued love and support while writing this book.

Second, I'd like to commend all of the people with hyperthyroid conditions who are open minded enough to look for a natural treatment solution.

Third, I'd like to commend all of the other healthcare professionals who use holistic treatment methods to help their patients.

I'd like to offer special thanks to Dr. Annette Schippel, who played a huge role in helping to restore my health back to normal when I was diagnosed with Graves' Disease.

Finally, I'd like to thank Dr. Janet Lang, whose protocols were used to help restore my health back to normal, and I currently use many of these protocols to help many people with hyperthyroidism and Graves' Disease.

Table of Contents

Why Natural Treatment Methods?

MANY PEOPLE WHO have hyperthyroidism or Graves' Disease might wonder why they should consider natural treatment methods. After all, if their endocrinologist or general medical practitioner has recommended antithyroid drugs or radioactive iodine therapy, then why question these conventional treatment methods? Since these doctors have been trained to help people with endocrine disorders it might seem to be foolish to attempt treating such a condition naturally.

Plus, most endocrinologists label hyperthyroidism and Graves' Disease as being incurable. Let's not forget we're talking about specialists who have received many years of training. So shouldn't they know better than some "wacky" holistic practitioner who claims that someone with a hyperthyroid condition can have their health restored back to normal through a natural treatment protocol?

While it might make complete sense to follow the advice of your medical doctor without considering alternative treatment methods, one needs to keep a few things in mind. First of all, the reason why most endocrinologists advise their patients with hyperthyroidism and Graves' Disease to take prescription drugs or receive radioactive iodine treatment is because this is how they have been trained. As you might have guessed, there is no holistic training class in medical school, as doctors are taught to treat most conditions through drugs, surgery, and other conventional methods. And the same concept applies with the endocrinologist specialty, as they go through extensive training to obtain these credentials, but they are taught to treat most hyperthyroid conditions with antithyroid medication, radioactive iodine, or thyroid surgery.

Of course there are times when conventional medical treatment is necessary. So I'm not suggesting that everyone with Graves' Disease or other types of hyperthyroidism shouldn't take antithyroid drugs, or receive radioactive iodine. Without question some people with hyperthyroid conditions do need to take medication to manage the symptoms, and some also will need to receive RAI. And sometimes even surgery is required. But the reason why I wrote this book is because while some people do need to receive conventional medical treatment, many people with primary hyperthyroidism and Graves' Disease can restore their health back to normal through natural treatment methods. And many people who can't have their health completely restored back to normal can still benefit from following a natural treatment protocol.

There Is No Official "Hyperthyroid Specialist"

While it's safe to say that many endocrinologists see a fair share of people with hyperthyroidism and Graves' Disease, they also focus on other endocrine disorders as well. This includes hypothyroidism and Hashimoto's Thyroiditis, diabetes, and numerous other endocrine disorders. This isn't to suggest that these doctors aren't competent with hyperthyroid conditions, but my point is that they have to deal with many different endocrine disorders, and as a result most don't have the time to look into holistic methods to help their patients. And to be frank, most of these doctors probably don't have the desire to use natural treatment methods on their patients.

Once again, these doctors simply aren't trained in medical school to treat any endocrine disorders naturally. So when someone comes into their office with a hyperthyroid condition, or any other endocrine disorder, they don't think to themselves, "what is the actual cause of this condition?" Instead, they will run their set of tests, and then based on the test results they will put the person on the necessary medical protocol. For diabetes, this frequently involves telling the person they will need to take insulin daily for the rest of their life, although they will also need to inform the person of modifying what they can eat and drink. For hypothyroidism, they will almost always recommend the patient to take synthetic thyroid hormone, rather than trying to find out why the person became hypothyroid to begin with (yes, natural treatment methods can benefit many of these people too!). And with hyperthyroidism and Graves' Disease, they will either have the patient take prescription drugs to put the condition into a state of remission, which is usually temporary, or they will right off the bat advise the patient to receive radioactive iodine treatment.

Why Not Find The Underlying Cause Of The Disorder?

On the other hand, many holistic doctors take the opposite approach. While they might order the same thyroid blood tests and recommend other similar tests, a good holistic doctor will also try to determine the cause of the condition. Because by looking into the cause of the disorder, many people with a hyperthyroid condition can have their health restored back to normal by addressing that cause. And as I have already mentioned, for those people who can't have their health restored back to normal, many can still receive some great benefits from natural treatment methods, and at the very least prevent their condition from worsening over time.

For example, it is agreed by numerous healthcare professionals that stress is a potential cause of hyperthyroidism and Graves' Disease. And while there is no definitive way to determine whether stress has caused someone's condition, one can get a good idea of whether stress is a factor by looking at the patient's history, and also by measuring the health of the patient's adrenal glands, which is almost never done by most medical doctors. And when they do recommend a test to determine the health of the adrenal glands, it is almost always a one-sample blood test of the morning cortisol levels, which in most cases isn't sufficient.

In any case, if it was determined that stress was a probable cause of someone's hyperthyroid condition, or at least a contributing factor, then one can help the patient to better cope with the stress in their life. Doing this alone probably wouldn't cure their hyperthyroid condition, but without question it is an important factor in restoring someone's health back to normal. And of course helping them cope with stress better can also prevent their condition from becoming worse over time.

The United States vs. Other Countries

The truth is that when compared to other countries, many medical doctors in the United States use invasive procedures on a more frequent basis. I'm not just talking about hyperthyroid conditions, but many other conditions as well. This would be fine if it led to a better outcome when compared to other countries, but this usually isn't the case. For example, the most common surgery in the United States is the Caesarean section, which no doubt can save lives in many pregnant women. But the C-

Section rate is much higher when compared to some other countries that have a much lower mortality rate. In other words, while some C-sections are without question necessary, many are done unnecessarily.

In fact, according to an article written in the New York Times, "The Caesarean section rate in the United States reached 32 percent in 2007, the country's highest rate ever".[1] A rate of around 15 percent would be ideal according to The World Health Organization. The article also states, "When needed, a Caesarean can save the mother and her child from injury or death, but most experts doubt that one in three women need surgery to give birth. Critics say the operation is being performed too often, needlessly exposing women and babies to the risks of major surgery."[2]

The same concept applies with the hysterectomy, as while this type of surgery is also necessary in some women, in many women this procedure is performed unnecessarily. Over 500,000 women receive this procedure each year. Don't get me wrong, as in the case of uterine cancer or other serious health issues, a hysterectomy may be warranted. But just as is the case with C-sections, many women receive a hysterectomy when there are alternative options.

According to Elizabeth Plourde, author of the book "Your Guide to Hysterectomy, Ovary Removal, & Hormone Replacement", "Though the first hysterectomies were implemented to save women's lives, now only 10% are the result of cancer, and less than 1% for obstetrical emergencies. The other, approximately 89%, are classified as "elective" surgery, and are performed for conditions that are not life-threatening.[3]

It's a similar situation with the thyroid gland. And one can argue that the thyroid gland is much more important than the uterus, or any other gland or organ frequently removed (gallbladder, appendix, etc.). While one can live without a uterus, gallbladder, tonsils, appendix, etc., nobody can live without a thyroid gland unless they take synthetic or natural thyroid hormone. So while nobody wants to have any gland or organ removed, one can argue that the thyroid gland is one of the LAST parts of the body you would want removed.

Try To Keep An Open Mind

In order to benefit from this book, it is important for you to keep an open mind. I of course don't expect you to agree with everything I say. In fact, I expect you to be skeptical. Just keep in mind that my goal isn't to convince you to choose natural treatment methods and avoid conventional medical treatment protocols. Instead, my goal is to show you the benefits of natural treatment methods, including how such treatment methods helped with my autoimmune hyperthyroid condition, and at the same time discuss the different benefits and risks of all of the different treatment options out there.

While I'm obviously biased towards natural treatment methods, I once again do realize that there is a time and place for conventional medical treatment, and I ultimately want to provide you with the information you need to make an informed decision. If after reading this book you decide to choose a natural treatment protocol then that's great. On the other hand, if you decide that conventional medical treatment methods are the best option for you, then that's fine too. But as long as you have explored all of your options and feel comfortable with your decision, then I'll feel as if I did my job.

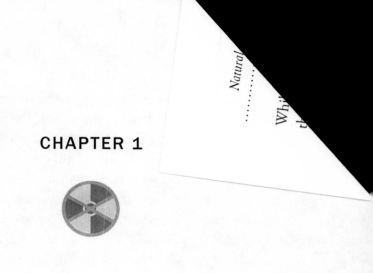

CHAPTER 1

What This Book Isn't About

THERE ARE NUMEROUS books out there about hyperthyroidism and Graves' Disease. Most of them go into great detail about the condition itself, giving a detailed explanation about how the thyroid gland works, the physiology of the endocrine system, the difference between T4 and T3, the different types of thyroid antibodies, etc. This book won't go into much detail with regards to the anatomy and physiology of the endocrine system, and also won't give a detailed breakdown of the different thyroid blood tests, thyroid antibodies, etc. If you want to know about the anatomy of the thyroid gland, receive a detailed breakdown of the different thyroid blood tests available, and to better understand the physiology, then there are two books I would recommend you reading:

Book #1: *Graves' Disease: A Practical Guide* by Elaine A. Moore and Lisa Moore

Book #2: *Living Well with Graves' Disease and Hyperthyroidism: What Your Doctor Doesn't Tell You...That You Need To Know* by Mary J. Shomon

le there are other resources on hyperthyroidism and Graves' Disease, nese two books are considered a "must-read" for people with these conditions. Both Mary Shomon and Elaine Moore have put together wonderful researched books which focus on these conditions. In fact, if you were recently diagnosed with hyperthyroidism or Graves' Disease then you might even want to read these books before you read my book. Not that they're prerequisites, as this book is basic enough for most people to understand. But for some people it's helpful to fully understand the basic anatomy and physiology as it pertains to hyperthyroidism and Graves' Disease, gain a greater knowledge of the different thyroid blood tests, etc, before trying to understand why natural treatment methods are so effective. Just to let you know, while I think these both are great books, this doesn't mean I agree with everything these authors discuss. There are some things I disagree with, which is perfectly fine, as I'm sure there are some topics I discuss in this book which they will disagree with as well.

What You Should Expect From Reading This Book

As I just mentioned, I try to keep this book very basic and easy to understand, as I don't go into great detail about the anatomy and physiology of the thyroid gland and endocrine system, and I talk about some of the conventional medical tests and treatments only on a basic level. The primary focus of this book is to show you how myself and other people with hyperthyroid conditions restored their health back to normal by following a natural treatment protocol, and how you can do the same.

A lot of the information in this book is based on my personal experience with Graves' Disease, as well as what I've seen by consulting with other people with hyperthyroid and autoimmune hyperthyroid conditions. While a lot of this information is based on the experience of myself and my patients, just like any book, at times I will make references to other sources as well. Although I did spend time doing research for this book, please keep in mind that there hasn't been much research with regards to natural treatment methods. This should be easy to understand when you realize that most research studies are actually set up by the pharmaceutical companies.

So while there are some references in this book, most of the information in this book is not based on hundreds of clinical studies on the effectiveness of natural treatment methods, but is instead based on my personal experience with Graves' Disease, the experience of my patients, and the fact that we were born with our thyroid gland for a reason. Truth to be told, we don't develop hyperthyroidism and Graves' Disease due to a deficiency of radioactive iodine, Methimazole, or PTU. This doesn't mean that people don't need these conventional medical treatment methods, but to tell everyone with hyperthyroid conditions to either take antithyroid drugs and pray for a remission, or to obliterate their thyroid gland using radioactive iodine is in my opinion ludicrous.

Despite the lack of research out there, once you are done reading this book I don't think you'll find it difficult to understand how natural treatment methods might be able to restore your health back to normal. The reason for this is because a lot of what I discuss is based on common sense. This of course doesn't mean that everyone with hyperthyroidism and Graves' Disease can have their health restored back to normal, but after reading this book you'll discover why most people with hyperthyroid conditions can greatly benefit from following a natural treatment protocol.

Here is a brief summary of the different chapters which are in this book:

Chapter 2: My Personal Story. In this chapter I discuss my personal experience with Graves' Disease, and how I was skeptical about whether holistic treatment methods would be able to restore my health back to normal. I also briefly discuss how I began helping people with thyroid and autoimmune thyroid conditions.

Chapter 3: Hyperthyroidism vs. Graves' Disease: What's The Difference?
In this chapter I discuss the difference between primary hyperthyroidism and Graves' Disease. The truth is that just about all of the information in this book can benefit people with any type of hyperthyroid condition.

Chapter 4: Finding The Underlying Cause Of Your Condition. In this chapter I discuss how most endocrinologists and other types of medical doctors don't look for the actual cause of the hyperthyroid condition. On the other hand, the goal of a competent natural endocrine doctor will be to find the underlying cause of your condition in an attempt to restore your health back to normal. This chapter will discuss some of the systems of the body which can lead to the development of hyperthyroidism or Graves' Disease.

Chapter 5: My True Feelings About Conventional Medical Treatment Methods. In this chapter I focus on conventional medical treatment methods. While many people might think I'm opposed to people taking antithyroid drugs and receiving radioactive iodine, the truth is that I realize there is a time and place for these types of treatments.

Chapter 6: Do Natural Treatment Methods Really Provide A Permanent Cure?
In this chapter I discuss whether natural treatment methods can provide a permanent cure for hyperthyroidism and Graves' Disease, or if they just provide a temporary solution.

Chapter 7: The Immune System Component Of Graves' Disease. In this chapter I discuss the importance of the immune system, and how conventional medical treatment does nothing to address the immune system component. I also discuss four factors which can lead to a compromised immune system.

Chapter 8: The Role That Stress Plays In The Development Of Graves' Disease. In this chapter I discuss how prolonged stress can potentially lead to the development of hyperthyroidism and Graves' Disease, and how stress affects the adrenal glands. I also list 12 stress management tips to help better manage your stress.

Chapter 9: The Importance Of Proper Digestion In Restoring Your Health Back To Normal. In this chapter I discuss why it's important to have a properly functioning digestive system for anyone looking to restore their health back to normal, and I give eight tips to help improve your digestive health.

Chapter 10: Hyperthyroid Diet Tips. In this chapter I give an actual "hyperthyroid diet" you can follow, and also reveal three important rules anyone with hyperthyroidism or Graves' Disease should follow.

Chapter 11: Nutritional Supplements and Herbs For Hyperthyroidism & Graves' Disease. In this chapter I discuss some of the nutritional supplements and herbal remedies which can help people with hyperthyroidism or Graves' Disease. I actually list some of the supplements and herbs I personally took initially during the natural treatment protocol I followed.

Chapter 12: The Truth About Iodine And Hyperthyroidism. In this chapter I talk about how many people with hyperthyroidism and Graves' Disease have an iodine deficiency. This is true even though many doctors recommend that people with hyperthyroid conditions avoid taking iodine. I also mention two methods to help determine whether someone has an iodine deficiency.

Chapter 13: Can Environmental Toxins Trigger Graves' Disease? In this chapter I discuss the impact of environmental toxins on our health, and how it can lead to an autoimmune thyroid disorder such as Graves' Disease. I focus on xenohormones, and explain how most people can do a better job of avoiding these toxins.

Chapter 14: How Big Of A Role Does Genetics Play? In this chapter I discuss how genetics alone doesn't determine whether someone will develop hyperthyroidism or Graves' Disease, and how environmental factors may play a greater role. I also discuss how to find out if you have a genetic marker for a thyroid condition.

Chapter 15: Graves' Disease & Thyroid Antibodies. In this chapter I discuss the significance of the tests for thyroid antibodies and whether a natural treatment protocol will help to lower these antibodies. I also talk about the radioactive iodine uptake test and whether or not it is really necessary for people with a hyperthyroid condition to receive this test.

Chapter 16: Why Radioactive Iodine Should Usually Be The Last Resort. In this chapter I discuss three reasons why radioactive iodine therapy usually should be the last resort. I also mention two primary situations when radioactive iodine therapy might truly be necessary.

Chapter 17: The Risks Of Playing The Waiting Game. In this chapter I discuss the risk of taking antithyroid drugs and hoping it will put you into a state of remission.

Chapter 18: Combining Natural Treatment Methods With Conventional Treatment Methods. In this chapter I discuss why it might be wise for some people to continue taking antithyroid medication while beginning a natural treatment protocol. I also discuss the herbs Bugleweed and Motherwort, and whether they can be safely used as substitutes for antithyroid drugs.

Chapter 19: Can Natural Treatment Methods Help With Thyroid Nodules? In this chapter I discuss how natural treatment methods might be able to help with thyroid nodules, but I also list four situations when someone with thyroid nodules might want to consider using medical intervention.

Chapter 20: Overcoming Thyroid Eye Disease. In this chapter I discuss how following a natural treatment protocol can potentially help someone who has thyroid eye disease.

Chapter 21: Natural Treatment Methods During Pregnancy & Lactation. In this chapter I discuss the different treatment options for women with hyperthyroidism and Graves' Disease who are pregnant or breastfeeding, including the risks involved with each of these treatment methods.

Chapter 22: Thyroid Storm & Natural Hyperthyroid Treatment Methods. In this chapter I discuss the condition known as thyroid storm, and whether or not natural treatment methods can help with this condition.

Chapter 23: 5 Reasons Why You Shouldn't Self-Treat Your Hyperthyroid Condition. In this chapter I discuss why people with hyperthyroidism and Graves' Disease shouldn't self treat their condition, giving five specific reasons. Many people look to treat their condition naturally, and if this describes you, then you definitely will want to read this chapter carefully.

Chapter 24: Natural Treatment Methods Don't Cure Anything. In this chapter I talk about how natural treatment methods don't cure hyperthyroidism or Graves' Disease, but instead strives to put the body into an optimal state of health.

Chapter 25: The Keys To Maintaining Your Health After Following A Natural Treatment Protocol. In this chapter I discuss how people who have restored their health back to normal need to maintain their health. I include six supplements I currently take to maintain a state of wellness.

Chapter 26: Consult With A Natural Endocrine Doctor. In this chapter I discuss the importance of speaking with a holistic doctor who focuses on endocrine disorders. I also give some advice when it comes to choosing a natural endocrine doctor.

Chapter 27: Formulate An Action Plan To Restore Your Health Back To Normal. In this chapter I discuss some things you can do right now to help restore your health back to normal.

Chapter 28: Your Number One Free Resource Center For Natural Thyroid Health. This chapter is a shameless self promotion of my website (www. GravesDiseaseBook.com), and essentially discusses the different areas of my website that you may find valuable.

Chapter 29: Twenty One Questions You May Have About Natural Treatment Methods. In this Chapter I answer twenty one of the common questions people have about natural treatment methods. Here are just a few of the questions I answer:

- Should Gluten Be Avoided In People With Hyperthyroidism & Graves' Disease?
- Can Natural Treatment Methods Help People With Subclinical Hyperthyroidism?
- Can Goiter Be Cured In People With Hyperthyroidism & Graves Disease?
- Can A Vegetarian Receive Good Results When Following A Natural Treatment Protocol?

Reading This Book Can Change Your Life

I have had many people email me after visiting my website, stating that the information I provided has changed their life. I'm hoping the same thing will happen after you read this book. In fact, a lot of the content which is on my website I also provide in this book. While I provide many articles, blog posts, and videos on my website, this book will provide you with some of the more important information you will need to help restore your health through natural treatment methods.

You should think of this book as an investment in your health, as not only can it help to restore your health with regards to your hyperthyroid condition, but it should also help with your overall health as well. With that being said, I would like to thank you for taking the time to read this book, and I'm confident that you find the following information to be extremely valuable.

CHAPTER 2

My Personal Story

SINCE GRADUATING FROM chiropractic college in 1999 I had considered myself to be in a good state of health. Although I didn't eat a perfect diet upon graduating, I think it's safe to say that I ate better than most people, exercised regularly, obtained at least seven to eight hours of sleep each night, etc. But one day I was walking into a retail store and saw one of those sit-down automated blood pressure machines. It had been a few months since I measured my blood pressure, and so I decided to get my blood pressure taken.

My blood pressure was fine, but I was shocked when the device revealed that my pulse rate was 90 beats per minute. Normally my pulse rate was in the mid 60's, and so I wasn't sure what was going on at the time. I immediately took my pulse rate manually, thinking that perhaps the machine wasn't working correctly. But sure enough, the manual readings were right around the same number.

The next few days I continued to monitor my pulse rate manually, and at any given time it was anywhere from 80 to 100 beats per minute. At the time I had also lost a lot of weight, but a few months before discovering the high pulse rate I followed a nutritional purification program and then continued eating well, and so I thought the weight loss might be due to my new regimen. It wasn't until after I discovered that I had a high pulse rate when I started linking this with the weight loss, and then I knew I had to get this checked out.

Off To The Medical Doctor I Went!

So I made a rare trip to a medical doctor, and after receiving the TSH and free T4 blood tests, I was told that I had a hyperthyroid condition. To be honest, I wasn't too concerned at the time, as I was relieved that I didn't have something more serious, such as cancer. On the other hand, being a holistic doctor I was familiar with hyperthyroidism, and I knew that radioactive iodine was commonly recommended by endocrinologists. Plus, as is the case with most people who have been diagnosed with any type of condition, I of course did plenty of research online.

So when I visited an endocrinologist about one month later I was prepared for her to recommend radioactive iodine to obliterate my thyroid gland. When I went to the endocrinologist, she performed some tests in the office, recommended other blood tests (free T3, tests for thyroid antibodies, etc.), and eventually diagnosed me with Graves' Disease. My goal here isn't to go into detail about the purpose of the different tests, as I mentioned in an earlier chapter that there are some good books out there which go into great detail about the radioactive iodine uptake test, thyroid blood tests, thyroid antibodies, etc. I will discuss some of these tests briefly in this book, but if you want this information in greater detail there are plenty of other resources out there which have this information.

Fortunately the endocrinologist I saw was somewhat conservative and to my surprise she just told me that I should take Methimazole and a beta blocker and hope my condition goes into remission. However, even before I saw this doctor I knew I was going to try following a natural treatment protocol. Being a holistic doctor, I knew that there had to be a cause behind my Graves' Disease condition, and I also knew that taking antithyroid drugs or receiving radioactive iodine treatment might help manage the hyperthyroid symptoms, but wouldn't do anything to address the cause.

Even I Was Skeptical About Holistic Treatments

Even though I'm a holistic doctor and made up my mind that I would follow a natural treatment protocol in an attempt to cure my Graves' Disease condition, this doesn't mean I wasn't skeptical. Without question I had my doubts about whether such a treatment protocol would restore my health back to normal. Quite frankly, I wasn't even looking for a complete cure, as I would have been happy with natural symptom management. I just wanted to avoid having to take prescription drugs, and definitely wanted to avoid receiving radioactive iodine.

At first I was planning to self-treat my condition. After all, I'm a holistic doctor, and while I didn't have much experience dealing with people who had hyperthyroid conditions at the time, in the past I did see a lot of people with hypothyroidism, fibromyalgia and other chronic conditions in my practice, and so I did wonder why I couldn't simply self-treat my condition? But after thinking it through, I decided to play it safe and I consulted with another holistic doctor who focused on endocrine disorders. And it turned out to be one of the best decisions I ever made.

The most annoying symptoms I had were the high pulse rate and palpitations I experienced, although I also had lost a lot of weight (I went from

180 pounds to around 140 pounds), and I had a voracious appetite. During the drawing of my thyroid blood tests I also experienced "shakiness", as when they drew the blood I found it difficult to keep my arm from shaking. After only a few weeks of following a natural treatment protocol I began noticing a decrease in the increased heart rate and palpitations. A few months later my palpitations were just about gone, my pulse rate normalized, the shakiness was gone, and I had gained a lot of the weight I lost back (fortunately not all of it!). The only symptom which remained was the voracious appetite, although this eventually disappeared as well.

As for the blood tests, a few months after beginning the natural treatment protocol my thyroid blood tests began to improve. There is no better feeling than the one I had when I received my first follow up blood tests and saw the improvement. Actually, there was a better feeling than this, as a few months later when I received another set of tests they had completely normalized. Overall it took about six months for my thyroid blood tests to become completely normal. I also received additional "alternative" tests which I will discuss in this book, and these tests also improved.

The Student Becomes The Teacher

After seeing how effective natural treatment methods were in helping with my autoimmune thyroid condition, I developed a passion to help other people with hyperthyroidism and Graves' Disease, as well as other thyroid and autoimmune thyroid conditions. After all, I knew there were thousands of people each year who had their thyroid gland obliterated through radioactive iodine treatment, and I felt that many of these people could be helped through natural treatment methods. The problem is that most people with hyperthyroidism and Graves' Disease aren't even aware that a natural treatment protocol might be able to help them.

I then began consulting with people who had primary hyperthyroidism, Graves' Disease, and other endocrine conditions who were interested in using natural treatment methods to restore their health back to normal. While there is no official certification for natural endocrinology (at least not yet), I learned a great deal by following a natural treatment protocol for my own hyperthyroid condition, and of course I have learned even more by helping others. Plus I also have attended numerous seminars and webinars on natural endocrinology, nutrition, etc. And since I began this venture I've been surprised as to how many people have expressed interest in using natural treatment methods to restore their health back to normal.

I also created a website called www.NaturalEndocrineSolutions.com. This website not only focuses on natural treatment solutions for hyperthyroidism and Graves' Disease, but other thyroid and autoimmune thyroid conditions. In addition, I created a guide entitled "The 6 Steps On How To Treat Graves' Disease and Hashimoto's Thyroiditis naturally", and offer this guide for free on my website. The guide contains some great content, and in addition to this guide I have created a lot of quality content on the website, as I write multiple articles and blog posts each week which inform people with hyperthyroidism, Graves' Disease, and other conditions as to how they can restore their health back to normal naturally.

Although I have thousands of people visiting my website each month, I still felt like there were many people with hyperthyroidism and Graves' Disease who weren't aware of the benefits of natural treatment methods. And so I decided to write this book, figuring a lot of people might not come across my website, but they just might discover my book and learn how a natural treatment protocol can possibly benefit them. I also created another website, www.GravesDiseaseBook.com, which focuses specifically on natural treatment solutions for hyperthyroidism and Graves'

Disease. This website also provides numerous articles and videos, and I actually modified the original free guide I created to make it specific to hyperthyroidism and Graves' Disease. So I would definitely recommend checking out this website as well. With that being said, let's move onto the next chapter and begin to discover how natural treatment methods might be able to restore your health back to normal.

CHAPTER 3

Hyperthyroidism vs. Graves' Disease: What's The Difference?

THROUGHOUT THIS BOOK you'll notice I keep on mentioning both "hyperthyroidism and Graves' Disease", rather than pertain to them both at the same time by simply saying "hyperthyroid conditions". Graves' Disease is the most common hyperthyroid condition. On the other hand, there are people with hyperthyroid conditions who don't have Graves' Disease.

What I'm basically doing in this book is separately referring to 1) hyperthyroid conditions without an autoimmune component, and 2) Graves' Disease, which is an autoimmune hyperthyroid condition. Of course one can't always completely rely on the tests which are routinely performed on people with hyperthyroidism. As a result, even if you have been diagnosed as having hyperthyroidism but not Graves' Disease, this doesn't mean you have a healthy immune system.

As a result, even if you have been diagnosed with hyperthyroidism and the tests for thyroid antibodies (TPO, TSI, etc.) were negative, as well as the radioactive iodine uptake test, all of the information in this book still applies to you as well, even the chapters which focus on "Graves' Disease". So yes, there are differences between primary hyperthyroidism and Graves' Disease, and other hyperthyroid conditions as well (i.e. toxic multinodular goiter, subclinical hyperthyroidism). But regardless of what type of hyperthyroid condition you have, I do strongly recommend that you read this entire book word for word, and not to skip over the chapters which focus primarily on Graves' Disease.

The same concept applies to my original website (www.NaturalEndo-crineSolutions.com), as if you visit it you will notice there are separate pages for "hyperthyroid conditions" and "Graves Disease". You'll also notice some articles I have written and videos I created focus on hyperthyroid conditions, while others focus on Graves' Disease. In most cases I do this for "niching and keyword purposes", as someone who has been diagnosed with Graves' Disease will find a headline with the word "Graves' Disease" more appealing than hyperthyroidism, while reverse is true with someone who has been diagnosed with primary hyperthyroidism. Similarly, when searching online, some people use the search terms "hyperthyroidism", while others use "Graves' Disease".

And just as is the case with my original website, with my other website, www.GravesDiseaseBook.com, there are different articles and videos which focus on "hyperthyroidism", and others which focus on "Graves' Disease". But once again, most of the content on this site will benefit people with any type of hyperthyroid condition.

In any case, whether you have primary hyperthyroidism or Graves' Disease, I expect you to find most of the information in this book to be valuable. And so even if you haven't been diagnosed with Graves' Disease, there is no guarantee that you won't develop it in the future. Because of this it's a good idea to read all of the information in this book which focuses on Graves' Disease and follow the advice given so you not only will restore your thyroid health back to normal, but you will also keep your immune system, adrenal glands, and other bodily systems healthy so that you hopefully will never develop an autoimmune thyroid disorder.

Chapter Summary

- Although most people with hyperthyroidism have Graves' Disease, there are different types of hyperthyroid conditions.
- Just because you haven't been diagnosed with Graves' Disease doesn't mean you have a healthy immune system. Many people who are diagnosed with primary hyperthyroidism will eventually develop Graves Disease.
- Whether you have primary hyperthyroidism, Graves' Disease, or another type of hyperthyroid condition, I expect you to find most of the information in this book to be useful.

For more information on these and other natural thyroid health topics, visit www.GravesDiseaseBook.com

CHAPTER 4

Finding The Underlying Cause
Of Your Condition

WHEN I FIRST began helping others with thyroid and autoimmune thyroid conditions, one of the first people I consulted with was a 29-year old female patient (we'll call her Rita) who developed hypothyroidism as a result of receiving radioactive iodine therapy. She was 22 years old when she made a routine visit to her medical doctor, and her blood tests revealed that she had hyperthyroidism, as she had low TSH levels. Even though she wasn't experiencing any symptoms at the time, she was referred to an endocrinologist, where it was recommended that she receive radioactive iodine treatment.

Like most people who are diagnosed with a hyperthyroid condition, Rita didn't know much about her condition. She also didn't realize the consequences of receiving radioactive iodine, and was convinced by the endocrinologist that this would be the best option to "cure" her condition. So even though she wasn't experiencing any symptoms at the time, she went ahead and received the radioactive iodine, and as a result had to take synthetic thyroid hormone on a daily basis to help manage the hypothyroid condition which eventually developed.

One thing which has puzzled me is how most endocrinologists and other types of medical doctors don't look for the underlying cause of hyperthyroidism and Graves' Disease. Whenever someone is diagnosed with a hyperthyroid condition, they are either told to 1) receive radioactive iodine to obliterate the thyroid gland, or 2) take antithyroid drugs and essentially pray that the condition goes into remission. Very rarely do they try to find the underlying cause and then attempt to cure this cause.

For example, it's no secret that everyone who has Graves' Disease has a compromised immune system. I know this, you know this, and your endocrinologist or general medical practitioner knows this as well. Yet, nothing is ever done to address the immune system component. Telling someone to receive radioactive iodine or to take antithyroid medication might help with the symptoms, but these treatment methods will do absolutely nothing for the immune system. Other bodily systems can be contributing to this condition as well, such as the adrenal glands, steroid hormones, and/or digestive system.

But these bodily systems are never looked at, as the focus is on the thyroid gland itself, which is rarely the direct cause of the condition. Sure, evaluating and treating the thyroid gland is important, but if one only focuses on the thyroid gland itself, then it shouldn't be a surprise why most endocrinologists label Graves' Disease as being incurable. Because the truth is that while conventional medical treatment is sometimes necessary for this autoimmune thyroid disorder, if the underlying cause isn't detected and then addressed, then one obviously won't be able to cure this condition.

What Causes These Other Bodily Systems To Malfunction?

Now you know that it's usually not the malfunctioning thyroid gland itself which is the root cause of the problem. One needs to look at the immune system, adrenal glands, steroid hormones, digestive system, and other areas of the body. But what exactly causes these other bodily systems to malfunction? I actually focus on some of the primary factors which can lead to this later on in this book, but for now let's briefly take a look at some of the factors which can compromise these bodily systems and lead to the development of hyperthyroidism, or an autoimmune thyroid disorder such as Graves' Disease.

Factor #1: An inability to handle stress. While most people know that stress can cause a lot of health problems, most don't truly understand the impact that chronic stress can have on one's health over a period of many months or years. The human body was designed to handle acute stress situations, but it can't effectively deal with prolonged, chronic stress. But it's not the chronic stress itself which causes the problem, but rather the inability to handle this type of stress.

So a person who deals with chronic stress and does a poor job of managing it will be more susceptible to developing these conditions when compared to someone who has better stress handling skills. The person with poor stress handling skills has a good chance of developing problems with their adrenal glands, which can affect immunity, digestion, as well as the thyroid gland itself. As a result, over a period of time a person with compromised adrenals can eventually develop an autoimmune thyroid condition, such as Graves' Disease. I'm not suggesting that this alone causes Graves' Disease, but I don't think it's a coincidence that most people with hyperthyroidism and Graves' Disease have problems with their adrenal glands.

Factor #2: Nutritional deficiencies. I believe that having one or more nutritional deficiencies can cause or contribute to conditions such as hyperthyroidism and Graves' Disease. And I'm not alone, as numerous other healthcare professionals agree with this. There are many different nutritional deficiencies one can have, and I'll discuss this in greater detail in another chapter.

Factor #3: Environmental toxins. I just mentioned earlier how it's impossible to completely eliminate the stress from your life. Similarly, it is also not likely that you will be able to avoid exposure to all of the environmental toxins. There are thousands of environmental toxins we're exposed to, and many of them are in the foods we eat and the products we buy. There's a book called "The Autoimmune Epidemic", which talks about how different environmental toxins can affect the immune system and possibly lead to the development of autoimmune conditions.[4] It makes sense when you think about it, as over the last few decades we have been exposed to more and more environmental toxins, and the rate of autoimmune thyroid conditions such as Graves' Disease have also increased. Obviously other factors are involved, but one can't overlook the impact of all the toxic chemicals we're constantly being exposed to on a daily basis.

Factor #4: Genetics. Although genetics can play a role in the development of primary hyperthyroidism, or an autoimmune condition such as Graves' Disease, the good news is that it does not play as big of a role as many people think. More and more studies show that people with genetic tendencies towards certain conditions may have such conditions triggered by external factors,[5] such as the three I just discussed. So rather than worry about whether your condition is caused by factors you can't control, you might as well focus on those factors which you do have control over.

So these are some of the common factors which can lead to the development of hyperthyroidism and Graves' Disease. Since most endocrinologists label these conditions as being incurable, it shouldn't surprise you that they don't focus on these factors, at least not the first three I mentioned. However, for a natural endocrine doctor, looking into these lifestyle factors is important when trying to restore the health of someone with a hyperthyroid condition.

Restoring The Health Of People With Hyperthyroidism And Graves' Disease Is No Easy Task

I do want to let you know that restoring the health of someone who has a hyperthyroid condition is not an easy process. Some people will try to self-treat their condition, but it really is a good idea to consult with a competent natural endocrine doctor, as such a doctor will look for the underlying cause of the problem. Once they determine the cause they will then put together an individualized natural treatment protocol to help restore the person's health back to normal.

This will no doubt include modifying some of the lifestyle factors I briefly discussed before. So if you do a poor job of managing the stress in your life, they will help you develop better stress handling skills. If nutritional deficiencies are the problem, then they obviously will encourage you to eat better, recommend the appropriate nutritional supplements, etc. With regards to environmental toxins, such a doctor will put you on a protocol to help eliminate many of these toxins from your body, and then educate you so you can continue to minimize your exposure to these toxins.

Being a natural healthcare professional, I'm of course biased, and therefore recommend that most people who have hyperthyroidism and Graves' Disease consult with a holistic doctor. After all, antithyroid drugs can be important to take on a temporary basis, but they don't do anything to address any of the factors I've discussed, and radioactive iodine therapy should usually be a last resort due to the damage it can cause to the thyroid gland. When you think about it, there really isn't much to lose by speaking with an expert, but there is a lot to potentially gain. Either way, in order for anyone with hyperthyroidism or Graves' Disease to restore their health back to normal they must take responsibility for their health.

Chapter Summary

- Most endocrinologists and other types of medical doctors don't look for the underlying cause of hyperthyroidism and Graves' Disease
- Conventional medical treatment methods typically do nothing for the underlying cause of the problem
- The malfunctioning thyroid gland itself usually isn't the root cause of the problem
- Other bodily systems such as the immune system, adrenal glands, steroid hormones, and digestive system usually cause or contribute to the development of the condition.
- Four factors which can cause these bodily systems to malfunction include 1) An inability to handle stress, 2) nutritional deficiencies, 3) environmental toxins, and 4) genetics.
- Restoring the health of someone who has a hyperthyroid condition is not an easy process

For more information on these and other natural thyroid health topics, visit www.GravesDiseaseBook.com

CHAPTER 5

My True Feelings About Conventional Medical Treatment Methods

SOME PEOPLE WILL no doubt perceive this book as a widespread criticism of conventional medicine. After all, this book focuses a great deal on how many people receive radioactive iodine unnecessarily, and how antithyroid drugs don't do anything for the cause of the hyperthyroid condition. Even though I do think that many people who choose conventional medical treatment methods can benefit from following a natural treatment protocol, I also realize that conventional medicine does have its place.

While some holistic doctors are strongly opposed to conventional medicine, I actually wish that both holistic doctors and medical doctors could work together, rather than fight one another. Without question there are a lot of things I don't agree with when it comes to conventional medical treatment, and the same thing can be said when it comes to how most medical doctors think of natural treatment methods. I don't think there's anything wrong with different types of doctors disagreeing with one another, but I do wish that more medical doctors would have an open mind towards alternative treatment methods.

My Feelings About The Pharmaceutical Companies

There is no question that prescription drugs save many lives, and that antithyroid drugs are important for many people with hyperthyroidism and Graves' Disease. On the other hand, many people take prescription drugs unnecessarily. So does this mean I'm opposed to the pharmaceutical companies? Although I definitely don't agree that drugs are the solution in most cases, they too have their place and are important at times. Plus, we also need to look at the business side of things.

The truth is that the pharmaceutical companies do a wonderful job of marketing their products both to medical doctors and to the consumer. In fact, many patients visit their medical doctor and ask for specific prescription drugs they see on television or read about on the Internet. This is perhaps the main reason why most people choose medical treatment methods, as we are being constantly inundated by print ads, commercials, and online advertising about these medications, while many people aren't even aware of the benefits of natural treatment methods. While the pharmaceutical companies do a great job of marketing their product, most holistic doctors don't do a good job of marketing alternative care.

Of course the same concept holds true with most medical doctors with regards to marketing their practices, as most medical doctors and holistic doctors don't know much about marketing their business, as their primary goal is to help patients. This of course is how it should be, although the fact is that to succeed in any business, marketing plays a very important role. The point I'm trying to make is that the success of the drug industry doesn't have much to do with the safety and effectiveness of prescription drugs, but instead can be credited to their astute marketing. Again, this isn't meant to criticize the industry, but is just meant to demonstrate what type of impact strong marketing can have.

The Role Of Credibility Factors In Choosing Conventional Medical Treatment

Of course credibility also plays a big role in people's decision to choose medical treatment over alternative care. As a whole, medical doctors are more credible than holistic doctors. Many people assume that because medical doctors go to medical school for many years and then spend many more years doing their residency that they have a greater amount of knowledge when compared to holistic doctors. I'm not arguing that most medical doctors are very knowledgeable in the field of medicine, but many holistic doctors receive an equivalent amount of training. For example, to become a chiropractor I received my bachelor's degree, spent an additional two years completing the prerequisite classes for chiropractic school, and then spent an additional four years in chiropractic college. The big difference is that most chiropractors complete their internship at the same time as taking their classes. In other words, during the last two years of school I took 24 credit hours per quarter and at the same time I was also required to see patients as part of my internship. On the other hand, medical doctors go through medical school and then complete their residency. So while both medical doctors and chiropractors obviously receive a different type of training, the duration is very similar. And the same concept holds true for some other holistic healthcare professionals, such as naturopathic physicians.

My goal isn't to take away any of the credibility of medical doctors, but it's to simply prove that many holistic doctors receive a sufficient amount of training as well. As I mentioned before, it would be great if more medical doctors and holistic doctors worked together, as this would benefit everyone. One thing it would accomplish is to give holistic doctors more credibility, although many people are already choosing alternative care over conventional medical treatment. But while I'm of course biased towards alternative treatment options, there are times when I do refer people to a medical doctor, and I do know that some medical doctors will recommend their patients to holistic doctors. The problem is that it's rare for this to happen, and so many people who can benefit from seeing an alternative doctor miss out because they aren't advised about natural treatment methods by their medical doctors. And the opposite holds true as well, as some people become turned off towards holistic doctors because some of these doctors try to cure every condition, and will never refer a patient to a medical doctor under any set of circumstances.

Do I see this pattern changing anytime soon? Definitely not, as while more medical doctors are becoming open minded towards alternative treatments, I still think it will be a long time before both medical doctors and holistic doctors work together on a regular basis.

Most People Are Looking For a "Quick Fix"

Even though our bodies have an amazing ability to heal, this takes time to happen, but most people are looking for a "quick fix" to their problem. There are some people who realize that prescription drugs are in many cases just covering up the symptoms, but they are fine with this. They don't have any interest in restoring their health back to normal. If their thyroid gland is malfunctioning, then they are perfectly fine with taking thyroid medication, even if it's on a permanent basis. If their cholesterol is high, then they see nothing wrong with taking statins (cholesterol-lowering medication) to provide a quick solution, rather than trying to get to the root cause of the problem. In other words, many people don't want to cure their condition, even when this is possible.

On the other hand, many people don't want to take drugs to manage their symptoms when they know there is the possibility of having their health restored back to normal naturally. Other people don't mind using medication such as antithyroid drugs on a temporary basis, but they still want to look for the underlying cause of the condition. This book is mainly aimed at these people. While I of course would love everyone with a hyperthyroid condition to read this book, the truth is that the only people who will read this book will be those who are open-minded towards alternative treatment methods. While more and more people are choosing natural treatment methods, there still are many who continue to choose conventional medical treatment methods due to many of the factors I discussed in this chapter.

Getting Medical Doctors To Open Their Minds Towards "Alternative Treatment Options" Is A Huge Challenge

While more and more consumers are choosing alternative healthcare, the same can be said about some medical doctors. Although most medical doctors still focus their practices on conventional medical treatments, some are becoming more aware of the benefits of alternative treatment methods. Part of this most likely has to do with them realizing that more and more of their patients are looking for alternative options. So even though medical doctors don't receive training in medical school about nutritional supplements and herbs, many people don't realize this, and so they will approach their medical doctor and ask them about the safety and effectiveness of certain supplements and herbs. As a result, some medical doctors are becoming more open minded and are attempting to learn more about some of the more common nutritional supplements and herbs being sold on the market.

As for whether it's feasible to change the opinion of medical doctors and to get them to realize the benefits of alternative healthcare, in most cases this will be extremely difficult to accomplish. It would of course give me great pleasure to have endocrinologists read this book and realize that there are other options besides antithyroid drugs and radioactive iodine. And while some endocrinologists and other types of medical doctors who read this will be open minded to the information presented in this book, I expect most medical doctors not to be receptive to this material. But then again, even if this book causes a few endocrinologists to change their approach when it comes to recommending antithyroid medication or RAI then this would be wonderful.

In summary, both conventional medicine and alternative healthcare has its place. And while it would be great if most medical and holistic doctors would work together, I don't see this happening anytime soon. Although more medical doctors are becoming receptive to alternative treatment methods, many medical doctors still remain opposed to holistic health-care.

Chapter Summary

- Although I think many people who choose conventional treatment methods would benefit from a natural treatment protocol, I also realize that conventional medicine has its place.
- Even though many people do need to take antithyroid drugs on a temporary basis, as well as other medication, many people take prescription drugs unnecessarily.
- Credibility plays a big role in people choosing medical doctors over holistic doctors, as most people perceive medical doctors as being more credible.
- Even though our bodies have an amazing ability to heal, it takes time for this to happen, but most people are looking for a "quick fix".
- While more and more people are turning towards alternative treatment methods, some medical doctors are also becoming more open minded towards alternative options.

For more information on these and other natural thyroid health topics, visit www.GravesDiseaseBook.com

CHAPTER 6

Do Natural Treatment Methods Provide A Permanent Cure?

WHEN CHARLIE WAS diagnosed with Graves' Disease, he was told by his endocrinologist to take Methimazole to help manage the symptoms. The plan was to have him take the medication for about 18 months, and hope that it would put him into a state of remission. Although some people respond well while taking the antithyroid drugs, Charlie just didn't feel good when taking the Methimazole. His endocrinologist recommended that he take PTU instead, which he did, but he still didn't feel right. Both medications did control the hyperthyroid symptoms, but he just didn't "feel like himself" while taking either one of them.

So Charlie decided to give natural treatment methods a try, and began noticing a big difference in the symptoms after about five weeks of following the protocol, and after three months his blood tests had dramatically improved, and he told me he felt the best that he had in years. Before beginning the natural treatment protocol Charlie ate a lot of refined foods and sugars, and didn't do a good job of managing his stress. During the protocol he ate much better, took certain supplements for additional nutritional support, and developed better stress handling skills.

However, once he started feeling great he began eating refined foods and sugars again (he did continue to do a good job of managing his stress). While this is fine when done in moderation after restoring one's health back to normal, he began eating these foods more and more frequently, and then one day he called me because he noticed his pulse rate was high again (although not as high as it was when he initially saw me), and he also began experiencing palpitations. He was upset because once the symptoms subsided he thought his condition was permanently cured, but as I tell everyone upon beginning a natural treatment protocol, "while I don't expect anyone to live a perfect lifestyle, if after restoring your health you neglect certain lifestyle factors there is a good chance you will suffer a relapse".

More Than Just "Natural" Symptom Management

When I talk about using natural treatment methods for hyperthyroidism and Graves' Disease, you may wonder if following such a treatment protocol can actually cure your condition, or will it just put your condition into a temporary state of remission? Before I answer this question, I first want to say that some people think of natural treatment methods as a "natural way" of managing the symptoms, and don't think of these treatment methods as doing anything for the actual cause of the disorder. I can tell you from experience that a genuine natural treatment protocol should do more than just naturally manage the symptoms, as you can of course just take prescription drugs for symptom management.

But as for whether natural treatment methods can actually cure hyperthyroidism, or an autoimmune thyroid condition such as Graves' Disease, I guess it's necessary to understand what the difference is between a cure and a state of remission. Most of us are familiar with a condition such as cancer being in a state of remission, and we understand cancer in remission as not actually being permanently cured, but instead the condition is under control and in a "dormant" state. In other words, someone who is in remission from a certain type of cancer still supposedly has the cancer, but it's not in its "active" form.

In fact, I have a friend who was diagnosed with a type of leukemia a number of years ago. He took a fairly new type of medication, and it not only controlled his symptoms, but over the last few years his leukemia has no longer been detectable on his blood tests. Despite this the doctors won't label him as being cured, but instead he has been told that he is in a state of remission. To put it another way, if he were to walk into another doctor's office who didn't know he was diagnosed with leukemia, they most likely wouldn't be able to tell he had such a condition, as all of the tests would come out negative. Yet, they consider this a state of remission and not a cure.

Let's look at another example. When someone has low back pain due to a pinched nerve and gets the problem resolved by seeing a chiropractor, is this person cured? Obviously this depends upon a number of different factors, such as what's causing the pinched nerve. But even if someone with a pinched nerve sees a chiropractor, receives treatment, and then it's determined that he or she is "cured", one can't argue that this person can suffer a "relapse" if they did the same things which originally caused the pinched nerve to develop in the first place. So if the pinched nerve was caused by lifting heavy objects on a frequent basis, combined with poor lifting techniques, there is a good chance the low back condition will "flare up" again if the person were to go back to this way of lifting.

What's The Difference Between A "Cure" And A "State Of Remission"?

When you think about it then, a cure really isn't much different than a state of remission. In fact, just about every condition which is cured can return, although there are certain exceptions. Of course the word "cure" is used rather loosely. For example, many endocrinologists consider radioactive iodine treatment as being a "cure" for hyperthyroidism and Graves' Disease. I've even read material which states that RAI is a cure for these conditions, and then goes on to mention how the person will need to take thyroid hormone daily for the rest of their life after receiving radioactive iodine. If you're talking about a permanent cure for the hyperthyroid symptoms then perhaps this is true. But this harsh treatment method is not actually curing the cause of the condition, as all it's doing is obliterating the thyroid gland in order to stop the hyperthyroid symptoms. So receiving radioactive iodine won't do anything for the underlying cause of the condition, as mentioned earlier in this book.

So do I consider my Graves' Disease condition as being permanently cured? I'd like to think so, as if I were to visit an endocrinologist and didn't tell them that I was previously diagnosed with Graves' Disease, and then went on to receive all of the standard testing (thyroid blood tests, tests for thyroid antibodies, etc.), then since all of these tests would come out negative they wouldn't label me as having Graves' Disease. But then again, these tests don't tell what the underlying cause of the condition is, and what's happening on a cellular level. So even if I received all of these tests and they came out negative, this wouldn't necessarily mean that I was cured.

As a result, one needs to look into some of the other "alternative" tests I received. For example, one such test I received was an Adrenal Stress Index test, which measures the levels of cortisol, as well as some other hormones (DHEA, 17-hydroxyprogesterone, etc.). This test actually did improve significantly after following a natural treatment protocol, as my depressed morning cortisol levels were within normal limits the last time I retested, and my DHEA also normalized after being depressed. However, even if some of the hormone levels on the ASI test were abnormal, it still wouldn't confirm that I had Graves' Disease. After all, many people who never have been diagnosed with Graves' Disease have weak adrenal glands, and therefore have low morning cortisol levels. Other people with Graves' Disease have high cortisol levels. In other words, having high or low cortisol levels and/or a low DHEA doesn't confirm the presence or absence of hyperthyroidism or Graves' Disease. However, many people with hyperthyroid conditions do have compromised adrenal glands and/ or a low DHEA.

The same thing can be said with other "alternative" tests as well. Let's look at another example involving a woman who was diagnosed with Graves' Disease and obtained a hair mineral analysis, which showed an imbalance of some of the trace minerals. This imbalance can be contributing to her Graves' Disease condition, but one can't definitively confirm this. In addition, it can take months to correct a single mineral imbalance, and so multiple imbalances can sometimes take years to correct. In any case, if this woman were to follow a natural treatment protocol and after six months had no hyperthyroid symptoms, and if all of the conventional medical tests to diagnose Graves' Disease were negative, but if she still had one or more mineral imbalances, could we then conclude that her Graves' Disease condition was cured, in a state of remission, or neither one?

The problem is that while alternative tests such as an Adrenal Stress Index test, male or female hormone panel, and hair mineral analysis test can help to determine some of the underlying factors of hyperthyroidism and Graves' Disease, one can't conclude that positive findings on any of these tests is in fact causing this condition. This of course doesn't mean they aren't important, as they are extremely valuable tests which provide important information for anyone with hyperthyroidism or Graves' Disease who is looking to restore their health back to normal. My overall point is that even though I sometimes use the word "cure" when talking about natural treatment methods, the truth is that there really is no way to determine whether someone is permanently cured, even if all conventional and alternative tests are negative. And if this is discouraging to you, hopefully reading the rest of this chapter (as well as the rest of this book) will convince you that it's still worth giving natural treatment methods a try.

A Relapse Is Always Possible

What you need to realize is that after following a natural treatment protocol, if you don't have any symptoms, if all of the conventional medical tests are negative, and if all of the alternative tests look great, this doesn't mean you're permanently cured. This doesn't just apply to hyperthyroidism and Graves' Disease, but most other conditions as well. For example, when I had my chiropractic practice in Concord, North Carolina, if a patient of mine had neck pain and then had their condition corrected through chiropractic adjustments, this doesn't mean the condition was permanently cured, as I eluded to earlier with the "pinched nerve" example. If this patient with the neck pain went and did the same things which caused the neck condition to develop in the first place, there is an excellent chance the neck pain would return. Similarly, if someone developed a cyst on their wrist due to some type of repetitive activity, and then had the cyst removed surgically, another cyst might develop if they kept stressing out the wrist.

With hyperthyroidism and Graves' Disease, it seems that lifestyle factors play a huge role in the development of these conditions, as I have already mentioned. Therefore, even if someone with a hyperthyroid condition has no symptoms and all negative tests, both medical and alternative in nature, this doesn't mean they can't suffer a relapse if they revert back to the same habits as before they followed a natural treatment protocol. So for example, if they ate plenty of refined foods and sugars and did a poor job of handling their stress before being diagnosed with Graves' Disease, and then upon following a natural treatment protocol they began eating well, improved their stress handling skills, and received the appropriate adrenal support, this definitely would help them with the recovery process. However, if after being "cured" they began eating junk food again and let stress get the best of them, a relapse would be likely to occur. It might take a few months, or even a few years before the condition returned, but there is an excellent chance this would happen.

Symptoms And Blood Tests Are Important, But...

While a person's symptoms and blood test results are important factors, the truth is that the body is very complex. As a result, just because someone is asymptomatic and all the tests are negative doesn't mean they don't have a condition, whether it be hyperthyroidism, Graves' Disease, or something else. After all, a person's symptoms is frequently the last thing to develop, which means that when a person develops a condition such as hyperthyroidism or Graves' Disease, it usually takes a long time until any symptoms are present. And by the time the blood tests are positive, the condition is also fully developed.

This is why it's important to look at alternative tests. But as I just mentioned before, these tests aren't specific for any condition. While there may be certain hormone and mineral imbalances someone with hyperthyroidism and Graves' Disease is likely to have, there is no specific "hyperthyroid hormone", or "Graves' Disease mineral". So while alternative tests can be extremely valuable, there is no specific alternative test to confirm the presence or absence of hyperthyroidism and Graves' Disease.

Let's Shoot For A "Permanent Remission"

Let's get back to the original question for this chapter, which is "do natural treatment methods really provide a permanent cure?" The truth is that I honestly don't know, and neither does any healthcare professional. While I'd like to consider my Graves' Disease condition as being permanently cured, I believe that if I went back to the previous lifestyle habits I followed before I was initially diagnosed that there is a good chance a relapse would occur.

With that being said, even if the best case scenario for someone who followed a natural treatment protocol involved them being in a permanent state of remission by maintaining a healthy lifestyle after restoring their health back to normal, then I'm guessing that most people would accept this. I know that as long as I am able to avoid receiving radioactive iodine treatment or avoid taking antithyroid drugs that I would be perfectly fine with this. So while I'd like to think that natural treatment methods can offer a permanent cure to hyperthyroidism and Graves' Disease, even a permanent state of remission would be fine with most people if it meant not having to rely on medication or having their thyroid gland obliterated.

Chapter Summary

- An effective natural treatment protocol should do more than just manage your symptoms.
- A cure really isn't much different than a state of remission, as most conditions which can be "cured" can return.
- In addition to the conventional thyroid blood tests, one should evaluate some of the "alternative" tests out there (Adrenal Stress Index, hormone panel, etc.)
- However, when these alternative tests are negative, this doesn't definitely confirm whether someone is permanently cured
- With hyperthyroidism and Graves' Disease, lifestyle factors play a huge role in the development of these conditions.
- Even if natural treatment methods don't provide a permanent cure, but can provide a permanent state of remission, I think most people would fine with this.

For more information on these and other natural thyroid health topics, visit www.GravesDiseaseBook.com

CHAPTER 7

The Immune System Component Of Graves' Disease

FOR THOSE PEOPLE with an autoimmune disorder such as Graves' Disease it is essential to address the immune system component before addressing the thyroid gland itself. While many people think of Graves' Disease as being a thyroid disorder, the truth is that this is a serious auto-immune condition. It puzzles me how most medical doctors neglect the immune system component, and focus primarily on the thyroid gland. After all, every endocrinologist and medical doctor knows that the immune system is compromised in Graves' Disease, and using antithyroid medication to suppress the production of thyroid hormone, or radioactive iodine to obliterate the thyroid gland won't do anything to help improve the health of the immune system.

It appears that people who have autoimmune disorders such as Graves' Disease and Hashimoto's Thyroiditis are more likely to develop other autoimmune conditions in the future, such as Rheumatoid Arthritis and Lupus. And when you think about it, this shouldn't be a surprise, as if most endocrinologists don't do anything to help address the immune system of their patients who have an autoimmune thyroid disorder, then their immune systems will of course remain in a compromised state, and they will therefore be more susceptible to other autoimmune conditions. While genetics can play an important role in developing one or more autoimmune conditions, it would seem obvious that if one doesn't do anything to improve the health of the immune system when someone is diagnosed with Graves' Disease, then that person will have a greater chance of developing other autoimmune conditions in the future.

For example, when I was initially diagnosed with Graves' Disease, the endocrinologist I consulted with recommended that I take Methimazole, along with a beta blocker. And even though I didn't take the medication, I respected the fact that she didn't recommend that I treat my condition with radioactive iodine (which I of course would have rejected anyway). But besides recommending the prescription drugs, she didn't recommend anything else which could have helped with my immune system and thus prevent future autoimmune conditions from developing. While there might not be any surefire method of preventing an autoimmune condition from developing, one can at least reduce their chances of developing such a condition by having a healthy immune system.

As you know, the goal of most medical doctors is to control your symptoms, and not necessarily address the cause of your condition. And don't get me wrong, as symptomatic relief is important, and sometimes taking prescription drugs is necessary. This is especially true with many cases of hyperthyroidism and Graves' Disease, as if a person has a very high heart rate, then they might need to take prescription medication for awhile to help control the symptoms, or else the condition can become life threatening. Once again, medical doctors are trained to manage the symptoms, and so I understand their approach when they tell someone with a hyperthyroid condition to take antithyroid drugs and/or a beta blocker. But I still wonder why they don't do anything to help the person improve the health of their immune system.

Can A Compromised Immune System Cause Graves' Disease To Develop?

Another thing to consider is that a compromised immune system can potentially cause your Graves' Disease condition to develop in the first place. It makes sense that someone who has a genetic marker for Graves' Disease and also has a weak and unhealthy immune system would be more likely to develop this condition when compared with someone who has the same genetic marker, but has a healthy immune system. So for a person who has a compromised immune system and over time develops Graves' Disease, giving them antithyroid drugs or radioactive iodine treatment without addressing the immune system component is ludicrous. But while a compromised immune system can be the cause of your condition, it's important to know what caused the immune system problem in the first place. As I'll discuss in the next chapter, compromised adrenal glands affect immunity, and many people have problems with their adrenal glands. So for many people, it's the compromised adrenal glands which is the problem, as this is causing issues with the immune system, thyroid gland, and other areas of the body.

In order to correct the immune system problem, you should be aware of some of the factors which can lead to it becoming compromised in the first place. And while there are a number of different factors which can lead to a compromised immune system, there are four primary ones which can play a major role. You'll notice that these are factors which are repeatedly brought up in this book, and the reason for this is because neglecting these lifestyle factors will affect many areas of the body, including the endocrine system, digestive system, cardiovascular system, and yes, the immune system.

So here are the four primary factors which can lead to a compromised immune system:

1. **Chronic stress.** As I'll discuss in detail in the next chapter, many people deal with chronic stress, which our bodies were not designed to handle. This chronic stress can and usually will affect the immune system and adrenals. And while a competent natural doctor will usually address these areas before focusing on the thyroid gland itself, it is just as important to help the person manage their stress in order to aid in their recovery. While there is no way you will ever completely eliminate the stress from your life, chances are you can do a much better job of coping with it, which will do wonders when trying to restore the health of your immune system.

2. **Poor nutrition.** Just as is the case with stress management, I can easily dedicate an entire book just talking about proper nutrition, and I'll be focusing a separate chapter on the importance of diet and nutrition. In any case, poor nutrition without question can compromise your immune system. And while taking quality nutritional supplements and/or herbal remedies can definitely assist in restoring the health of your immune system, supplements are no substitute for eating well. Just about everyone needs to eat better, but in addition to eating well, most people will need to take some quality supplements so they can get the nutrients they aren't getting from their food. As you probably know, most people don't get all of the nutrients from the foods they eat, which is why everyone should at least take some basic nutritional supplements each day.

3. **Sleep deprivation.** This of course can go either way, as sometimes a person has no problem obtaining quality sleep until they acquire an autoimmune thyroid disorder. Then once they have the autoimmune disorder they begin having sleeping difficulties. On the other hand, some people who are healthy will neglect their sleep for a period of months, or even years, which can eventually lead to numerous health problems.

For example, some people who work a typical 8 to 5 shift will stay up late each night, and will end up averaging only 5 or 6 hours of quality sleep on a nightly basis. Over time, this can definitely have a negative impact on their immune system. On the other hand, people who work odd shifts which affect their sleep patterns can also be affected. Then there are people with an entrepreneurial background who spend countless hours on their business, getting up early in the morning and going to sleep late. This routine, combined with the stress of owning one's business, will almost definitely have a profound impact on their immune system. This type of work ethic also applies to many people working in the corporate world, as many people spend sixty or more hours per week on their job, and end up neglecting their health.

4. **Environmental toxins.** Someone can eat well, get ample sleep, and do a great job of managing stress, yet can still acquire a compromised immune system if they are constantly being exposed to environmental toxins, such as certain household cleaners and other products which emit dangerous chemicals. There are other types of environmental toxins as well, and while it is impossible to avoid them completely, most people can do a better job of reducing their exposure to such toxins. I'll discuss this in another chapter.

Is The Immune System Weak Or Is It Overactive?

With regards to Graves' Disease, I frequently talk about a "compromised" immune system, but what exactly does this mean? Does it mean the immune system is in a weakened state? Or does it refer to an overactive state? It's really a combination of both, although when I talk about strengthening the immune system in someone with Graves' Disease, many people will argue that you don't want to take this approach. They argue that you want to "calm down" the immune system. The goal of an effective natural treatment protocol is to do both, as strengthening the immune system doesn't mean that you're "boosting" it, or exacerbating the autoimmune response. It is necessary to address the autoimmune response, which is the overactive component, but at the same time you want the immune system to be healthy and strong.

To clarify this, if someone has certain deficiencies, such as low Vitamin D levels and/or low selenium levels, then one can argue that their immune system is in a weakened state. On the other hand, if this person also has high thyroid antibodies, then this would be considered to be an overactive state. So in this example, the goal of an effective natural treatment protocol would be to increase the Vitamin D and selenium levels to "strengthen" the immune system, and at the same time lower the thyroid antibodies.

In summary, if you have been diagnosed with an autoimmune thyroid condition, make sure you do what is necessary to restore the health of your immune system. You can of course try speaking with your endocrinologist or general medical practitioner about how to go about doing this, but as you know, most medical doctors don't receive adequate training in preventative care, which is why you'll see me constantly recommend that people with these conditions speak with a competent holistic doctor. Because if you don't address the immune system component of

Graves' Disease, then it won't be possible to restore your health back to normal.

Chapter Summary

- For people with Graves' Disease, it's important to address the immune system component before addressing the actual thyroid gland.
- Research has shown that people who have autoimmune disorders such as Graves' Disease are more likely to acquire additional autoimmune conditions in the future, such as Rheumatoid Arthritis and Lupus.
- While it can be important to take antithyroid drugs, they do nothing for the compromised immune system.
- Four factors which can lead to a compromised immune system include: 1) chronic stress, 2) poor nutrition, 3) sleep deprivation, and 4) environmental toxins

For more information on these and other natural thyroid health topics, visit www.GravesDiseaseBook.com

CHAPTER 8

The Role That Stress Plays In The Development Of A Hyperthyroid Condition

As I BRIEFLY mentioned earlier in this book, stress can play a role in the development of hyperthyroidism and Graves' Disease. I spoke about how chronic stress can weaken the adrenal glands, and in this chapter I'm going to go into greater detail about this.

I believe that chronic stress was a big factor in the development of my Graves' Disease condition. Although I'm sure there were other factors as well, I definitely dealt with a lot of chronic stress for many years. Obviously a lot of people deal with chronic stress, and it's not just the stress itself which is the culprit, but it's the person's ability to handle the stress which is a big factor. And I admittedly didn't do a good job of managing my stress.

First of all it's important to understand that the human body wasn't designed to handle chronic stress. The adrenal glands were designed to handle acute stress situations without much of a problem. But in today's world most people are overwhelmed with chronic stress, as they have stressful jobs, stressful relationships, financial problems, and many other stressful issues. And even though stress is common, most people don't do a good job of managing the stress in their life, as I just mentioned before.

Since the adrenal glands weren't designed to handle chronic stress situations, for a person who deals with a lot of stress AND does a poor job of managing it, what frequently happens is over a period of months and years there is an excellent chance their adrenal glands will weaken, which can eventually lead to adrenal fatigue. But even before reaching the point of adrenal fatigue, compromised adrenal glands can create other problems, including malfunctioning of the thyroid gland.

How Stressed Out Adrenal Glands Can Affect The Thyroid Gland

I originally learned how compromised adrenal glands can cause the development of a thyroid condition from Dr. Janet Lang, who like myself is a chiropractor who focuses on endocrine disorders. She has discussed how when the adrenal glands are stressed out, this puts the body into a state of catabolism, which means that the body is breaking down. Because of this, the body will slow down the thyroid gland as a protective mechanism. The reason behind this is because the thyroid gland controls the metabolism of the body, and so the body slows the thyroid gland down in order to slow down the catabolic process. This is why many times the thyroid gland won't respond to treatment until you address the adrenal glands.

While a hypothyroid condition is commonly caused by problems with the adrenal glands, this doesn't mean that compromised adrenal glands also aren't common in people with hyperthyroidism and Graves' Disease. In fact, many people, regardless of what type of thyroid or autoimmune thyroid condition they have, will have adrenal gland problems. But if people with compromised adrenal glands primarily develop hypothyroidism, why do some people with stressed out adrenals develop a hyperthyroid condition? I'm honestly not sure why this is the case, and I'm also not so sure that having weak adrenal glands alone directly causes hyperthyroidism to occur, but it definitely seems to be a contributing factor in many people with hyperthyroidism and Graves' Disease. Genetics could play a role in this, but there can be other factors as well. Either way, in my experience, in order to restore the health of someone with hyperthyroidism and Graves' Disease, it is necessary for that person to have healthy and strong adrenal glands.

Part of the reason behind this is because compromised adrenal glands cannot only affect the thyroid gland, but can also affect other areas of the body as well. Compromised adrenal glands can also affect the immune system, as well as the digestive system. In fact, here is what Dr. James Wilson, author of the well know book "Adrenal Fatigue" has to say about how the adrenal glands affect the immune system:

"When cortisol is elevated during an alarm reaction, there is almost a complete disappearance of lymphocytes from the blood. That is why your immune system is suppressed when you are under stress or taking corticosteroids. On the other hand when circulating cortisol is low, its moderating effect on immune reactions is lost and lymphocytes circulate in excess. In this situation inflammation is greater with more redness and swelling, and it takes a longer time for the inflamed tissue to return to normal. So, directly and indirectly cortisol dramatically influences most aspects of immune function".[6]

Donna Jackson Nakazawa, who is the author of the book "The Autoimmune Epidemic", also reveals how cortisol affects immunity:

> *"Prolonged levels of heightened cortisol can not only lead to an underfunctioning immune system, but can also indirectly stimulate an autoimmune response. Cortisol helps to regulate our immune-system response not only by turning on the immune response, but also by turning it off. When cortisol keeps being pumped out because of daily anxieties and stressors, we stop producing sufficient cortisol to signal the immune response to turn off. This increases the likelihood that the immune system will go into erratic overdrive, that mistakes will be made and autoantibodies will attack the body itself".*[7]

So while it's not known exactly why people develop hyperthyroidism and Graves' Disease, we do know that Graves' Disease is a hyperthyroid condition which involves a compromised immune system. And since the adrenal glands affect both the thyroid gland and the immune system, it makes sense to do what is necessary to restore the health of the adrenal glands back to normal.

One study of people with Graves' Disease suggested that major life events was a factor in the development of a hyperthyroid condition, and that "coping strategies" may help to improve the prognosis in people with Graves' Disease.[8] This study didn't conclude that stress was the main cause of Graves' Disease, and I'm definitely not suggesting that stress is the primary cause of this or any other hyperthyroid condition, but it does seem as if stress can play a huge role in the development of a hyperthyroid disorder.

Most Medical Doctors Don't Do Anything For Compromised Adrenal Glands

In the previous chapter I discussed how most medical doctors don't do anything to address the immune system component. This is true even though every endocrinologist and medical doctor knows that the immune system is compromised in Graves' Disease. So it shouldn't surprise you that most endocrinologists don't do anything to address the adrenal glands either.

Because in order to do this they would first need to determine whether someone has compromised adrenal glands to begin with, which most medical doctors almost never do. I take that back, as if they suspect a person has a severe adrenal condition such as Addison's Disease, then they will take a look at their morning cortisol levels and run other tests. But even though many people have compromised adrenal glands which can lead to numerous health issues, they usually don't do anything about this unless the person has a severe condition such as Addison's Disease. And once again, this is due to the training they receive in medical school.

Once again, my goal here isn't' to bash the medical profession. I just want to make you aware of this, so that you can understand yet another difference between visiting an endocrinologist and seeing a holistic doctor who focuses on endocrine disorders.

How To Determine Whether Someone Has A Problem With Their Adrenal Glands

One of the best methods of determining whether someone has compromised adrenal glands is through an Adrenal Stress Index (ASI) test. This is a saliva-based test by the company Diagnos-Techs, and involves the person taking four different saliva samples at different intervals throughout the day, which correlate with the circadian pattern. This is far more valuable than a single cortisol sample, which many doctors will take. Some doctors will take a single cortisol sample in the morning, and if it's low, they will determine that the person has a problem with their adrenal glands. This might be true, but it's best to look at the cortisol levels throughout the day.

This is especially important for someone who has high cortisol levels, which isn't uncommon. People with high cortisol levels will need to follow a completely different protocol than those with low cortisol levels. And in these people it is essential to know whether they have high cortisol levels not only in the morning, but at other points throughout the day as well. In fact, I've consulted with patients who had normal or low cortisol levels in the morning, but had high cortisol levels later in the day. So once again, just obtaining a one sample cortisol test in the morning isn't sufficient.

A Breakdown of The Adrenal Stress Index Test

Let's take a look at what the ASI test measures:

Cortisol levels: This is the primary hormone most holistic doctors will look at on this test, as this test will measure four different cortisol levels throughout the day to determine if you have a proper circadian pattern. Normally the cortisol levels should be at the highest levels in the morning upon waking up, and will decrease throughout the day. This pattern will help to give you the energy you need throughout the day, and the lower cortisol levels at night will allow you to fall asleep. These patterns will differ for someone who works odd shifts.

People with weak adrenal glands commonly have low cortisol levels in the morning. This was true when I had this test done after being diagnosed with Graves' Disease, as while I didn't feel like I had adrenal problems, the low cortisol levels on this test confirmed that I did in fact have weak adrenal glands. And if I didn't take the necessary steps to correct this, then over time the condition would have worsened, and most likely would have developed into "full blown" adrenal fatigue.

DHEA/DHEA-S: DHEA is manufactured by the adrenal glands, and plays a big role in immunity and in the stress response. DHEAS is the sulfated version of DHEA. If someone deals with chronic stress on a regular basis, this will also weaken the adrenal glands, and chances are these hormone levels will be low.

17-OH Progesterone: A steroid hormone that is a precursor to cortisol. This hormone is mainly produced in the adrenal glands (although it is also produced to some extent in the gonads), and because of this, when someone has weak adrenal glands these hormone levels will also typically be low.

Gliadin AB: This measures your sensitivity to gluten, which many people are allergic to. Consuming gluten when you're allergic to it can cause a lot of problems, not only with the digestive system, but also with adrenal health. One does need to be cautious however, as this test may not be completely accurate in someone with a compromised immune system. As a result, I don't rely on this test when it comes to people who have Graves' Disease, as well as other autoimmune conditions.

Secretory IgA: An antibody found in the saliva which plays an important role in immunity. Low values can indicate a problem with your immune system, which is common with people who have compromised adrenal glands.

...uw van You Tell If You Would Benefit From Adrenal Testing?

If you're consulting with a natural endocrine doctor, or any good holistic doctor, they will have you complete a detailed case history which will help determine if you have problems with your adrenal glands. Some of the more common symptoms include a feeling of exhaustion, sugar cravings, sleep disturbances, and there are many other symptoms one can have. Assuming you have at least some of these symptoms, there is a good chance the doctor will recommend a test to determine the health of your adrenal glands. There are companies other than Diagnos-Techs which offer adrenal testing, but this is the company I personally use, and I have had a great experience with them so far.

While I don't recommend self-treating adrenal fatigue, upon being diagnosed by a competent holistic doctor you can take some basic steps to help restore your health back to normal. If you read the book "Adrenal Fatigue, the 21st Century Syndrome" by Dr. James Wilson, he includes some detailed questionnaires to help determine if you have problems with your adrenal glands. Once again, you can't rely on symptoms alone, but I do think the questionnaires have some value and are worth checking out.

How To Restore The Health Of The Adrenal Glands

In order to restore the health of the adrenal glands, one obviously needs to address the cause of the problem. With regards to stress, it of course is impossible to eliminate all of the stress from your life. On the other hand, there are two things you can do when it comes to dealing with chronic stress which will lead to better health:

1. **Minimize the number of stressful situations.** Once again, you won't be able to eliminate all of the stress in your life, but in many cases it is

possible to reduce some of the stressful situations you are dealing with. Write down all of the different things in your life that you consider to be stressful, and try to figure out how you can make some changes to make things less stressful.

2. **Learn how to better cope with the stress in your life.** While it might be difficult to eliminate some of the stressful situations in your life, you do need to learn how to do a good job of managing stress. Of course there are many different ways to manage stress, as one can exercise or do yoga, get a relaxation massage every now and then, have a counseling session, eat a healthier diet, get more sleep each night, etc. These obviously are just a handful of basic examples, but I think you get the picture.

12 Stress Management Tips You Can Follow:

While the goal of this book isn't to get into detail about stress management, in a previous article on my website I discussed twelve stress management tips to help restore someone's thyroid health back to normal. So I thought it would be a good idea to include them here:

Tip #1: Try to keep a positive attitude most of the time. While a positive attitude alone isn't enough to manage your stress, having one can definitely help. Obviously nobody can be positive 100% of the time. But many people seem to always carry a negative attitude with them, which definitely won't help you cope with the stress in your life.

Tip #2: Begin a regular exercise program. You want to engage in some type of cardiovascular activity at least 3-4 times each week, ideally for at least 30 minutes each time. This can include taking a walk outside or on a treadmill, going on the elliptical machine or stationary bike, or anything else that will make you sweat a little. I realize some people with hyperthyroidism and Graves' Disease might not have the energy to exercise. If this describes you, even 20 to 30 minutes of walking will be beneficial. Besides engaging in cardiovascular exercise, other activities that can help you to manage stress include yoga and Pilates. Of course if you haven't exercised for awhile you do need to start out slow, and it's also wise to consult with your medical doctor first.

Tip #3: Eat healthier foods. Most of us can do a much better job of incorporating healthier foods into our diets. I don't expect anyone who has been eating poorly to immediately give up all of the "bad foods" they love. But even making small changes in what you eat can have a big impact on your health.

Tip #4: Drink plenty of purified water each day. Many sources suggest that you should drink at least eight tall glasses of water each day. The problem with this is that everyone has different needs based on their weight, and so I recommend that you should drink half of your body weight in ounces per day. So for example, if you weigh 140 pounds, then you would want to drink at least 70 ounces of water each day. And please don't drink tap water, as you really should be drinking purified water.

Tip #5: Take quality nutritional supplements. Since most of us don't eat a perfect diet, it's important to take some quality nutritional supplements on a daily basis. At the very least you should take a quality whole food multi-mineral vitamin and fatty acid each day. There are a lot of poor-absorbing supplements being sold, and so you do need to be careful. I personally recommend whole food supplements to my patients, rather than the synthetic vitamins which are sold by most retailers.

Tip #6: Get at least eight hours of quality sleep each night. I know this might be difficult to do, especially if you need to wake up early for work. And once again, some people with hyperthyroidism or Graves' Disease will have difficulty falling to sleep and/or will wake up in the middle of the night. So until they get this problem addressed then it admittedly will be difficult for them to get eight hours of quality sleep on a regular basis. Often times sleep problems are caused by stressed out adrenal glands, which most endocrinologists and medical doctors don't address.

Tip #7: Avoid environmental toxins as much as possible. While it's not possible to avoid these completely, you need to realize that these toxins really do affect your health. I'm not going to discuss everything you can do to avoid these toxins here, but I will tell you two things you can do to that will help you in the long term. First of all, install a filter in your shower that removes chlorine, as this can really help to boost your energy levels. Second, stop buying household cleaners with harsh chemicals, and instead get some natural household cleaners at your local health food store.

Tip #8: Make love more often. Having sex increases the endorphins in your body, which also will help you to manage stress. So make love with your partner more often.

Tip #9: Get a monthly massage. Schedule an appointment with a licensed massage therapist and treat yourself to a monthly massage. Massage therapy is not just about stress management, as there are many other benefits as well. But one of the big benefits of massage therapy is that it can help to relieve stress.

Tip #10: Consider seeing a chiropractor. Okay, I'm admittedly a little bit biased here, being that I have a chiropractic background. But since spinal adjustments help to balance out the nervous system, receiving them from a chiropractor can also help to relieve stress. Like massage therapy, there are so many other benefits when it comes to chiropractic.

Tip #11: Talk to someone. Sometimes speaking with someone can help relieve your stress. This doesn't necessarily mean talking with a counselor, although in some cases this can be helpful. But even talking with a good friend, family member, or acquaintance can really help.

Tip #12: Don't take life so seriously. This doesn't mean that you shouldn't take certain aspects of your life seriously. But on the other hand, many of us let things stress us out that really shouldn't. Write down a list of some of the things which cause stress in your life, and then take a look at these tips I have just given you, and determine how you can apply this advice to those things that stress you out on a regular basis.

For example, if you have a job that stresses you out, then perhaps you need to change your attitude (or change your job!). Or it might be that you're not eating well and/or not getting enough sleep. These lifestyle changes won't get rid of the stress in your life, but will help you better manage it. If your spouse is stressing you out, then perhaps counseling is the answer for you.

So here you have it, as if you follow at least 75% of these tips (9 of 12), including all of the first six I listed, you will do wonders in managing your stress. This admittedly is an incomplete list, as there are other things you can do to manage your stress. But these are some of the more important ones that can truly help to restore your health, and help you to maintain your health.

What If You Have High Energy Levels?

Just because someone has weak adrenal glands doesn't mean they will have low energy levels. Although this is common, some people with hyperthyroidism have weak adrenal glands, yet have high energy levels. When this happens it's usually in the beginning phases of the condition, not too long after a person has become symptomatic. I personally felt great from an energy standpoint immediately after being diagnosed with Graves' Disease, yet the Adrenal Stress Index test showed that I had low cortisol levels. I have consulted with other people with hyperthyroidism and Graves' Disease who also had a lot of energy months after being diagnosed, and didn't feel fatigued, yet also had weakened adrenal glands.

It once again is important to understand that it usually takes many years for the adrenal glands to become compromised. And once they become compromised, it then usually takes time for a person to become symptomatic. Some people develop fatigue quicker than others, but eventually any person with weakened adrenal glands will develop lower energy levels. So you can't rely on symptoms alone, and therefore we can't assume that someone who has high energy levels has perfectly healthy adrenal glands.

In summary, chronic stress can cause a lot of different problems, and if not managed it will affect the adrenal glands, which in turn can ultimately cause or contribute to hyperthyroidism or Graves' Disease. Of course this doesn't mean that all hyperthyroid conditions are caused by stress, but there's no question that stress is the culprit in many cases. And for those who have a hyperthyroid condition which was caused by stress, doing a better job of managing the stress in their life is essential if they want to use natural thyroid treatment methods to restore their health back to normal. But even for those who choose conventional medical treatments, it still will benefit your overall health to become an expert in stress management.

Chapter Summary

- Prolonged stress can be a big factor in the development of hyperthyroidism and Graves' Disease.
- Weak adrenal glands can potentially lead to the development of hyperthyroidism and Graves' Disease.
- An Adrenal Stress Index test can help determine whether someone has a problem with their adrenals.
- In order to restore the health of the adrenal glands, one obviously needs to determine what caused the problem with their adrenal glands in the first place.
- Reading the 12 stress management tips Iisted in this chapter will help you to better manage your stress, which in turn will help with your adrenal health.

For more information on these and other natural thyroid health topics, visit www.GravesDiseaseBook.com

CHAPTER 9

The Importance Of Proper Digestion In Restoring Your Health Back To Normal

UPON REVIEWING THE case history of "Rachel", I noticed that she had numerous symptoms which indicated less than optimal digestive health. She experienced frequent bloating and gas, had indigestion frequently, and she didn't have a daily bowel movement. As a result, one of the primary areas I needed to address was restoring her digestive health. A big part of this involved dramatic changes in her eating habits, as she had a horrible diet. Just as I tell many of my patients, I told Rachel that I didn't expect her to make these changes immediately, and so I told her to slowly begin incorporating more whole foods into her diet, and to greatly minimize the refined foods and sugars.

She had some pretty strong sweet and carbohydrate cravings, but when I recommended the herb Gymnema to help with her cravings, she decided she didn't want to take it. I told her this would be fine, as we can try to accomplish this without the Gymnema, as not everyone needs to take this. To make a long story short, after a few weeks Rachel said she was eating well, and so she began a natural treatment protocol. A couple of months went by, and she wasn't receiving the results we both had hoped for. After some probing she finally admitted that she still wasn't eating well, as she continued to eat junk food on a daily basis.

She realized that in order to have any chance of restoring her health back to normal she would have to make these changes. So she set a goal for two weeks where at that time she would be eating only whole foods. It wasn't easy, and she eventually did need the help of the Gymnema to control her cravings, but it she was able to change her diet, and it wasn't too long before she began experiencing an improvement in her digestive symptoms (along with many of her other symptoms), followed by some positive changes in her thyroid blood tests and antibody levels. But I'm pretty sure she wouldn't have reached this point if she continued eating refined foods and sugars numerous times each day.

Don't Overlook The Importance Of Having A Healthy Digestive System

When it comes to restoring one's health back to normal after being diagnosed with primary hyperthyroidism or Graves' Disease, one of the most important factors is how well you digest your food. In the next few chapters I will focus a great deal on eating well and the importance of proper nutritional supplementation. In fact, if you read any book that focuses on natural treatment methods for a specific condition, chances are it will discuss in detail how you need to eat well and take quality nutritional supplements.

However, eating quality foods and taking nutritional supplements won't do you much good if you aren't properly digesting what you consume.

Many people's digestive systems are so screwed up that their body does a poor job of digesting the food they eat and the supplements they take, which means they won't benefit much from them. This is yet another reason why someone who has been eating junk food on a daily basis for many years usually can't get well simply by changing their diet and taking supplements.

The Dangers Of Acid-Stopping Medication

Millions of people take acid-stopping medication, which in many cases just further impairs their digestive system, and thus interferes with their ability to digest the food they eat. Let's just think about this for a minute. One needs a good amount of acid in their stomach to digest the food they eat and any nutritional supplements they take. So if you take drugs which reduce the production of acid then there is no way you can properly digest the food and supplements you ingest. Of course if you have an excessive amount of stomach acid then perhaps these drugs can help (although they of course won't get to the underlying cause of the problem). But many people are told to take acid-stopping medication based solely on the symptoms they are experiencing, without confirming whether or not they truly have an excessive amount of stomach acid being produced.

Is it wise to take acid-stopping medication if you experience a lot of stomach burning and/or acid reflux? This isn't always due to an increase in the amount of acid, as it can be due to a decrease in the lining of your stomach due to poor eating habits, increased stress, and other lifestyle factors. And even when such symptoms are caused by an increase in stomach acid, the goal still should be to get to the cause of the problem. So yes, taking acid-stopping medication may help to manage the symptoms, but they will do absolutely nothing for the underlying cause of the problem. And the long term side effects it can have on your digestive system and your entire body can be disastrous.

It Takes Awhile To Fix Digestive Issues

As I just mentioned, beginning to eat well and taking quality supplements alone after years of eating junk food usually won't be enough to correct a digestive problem. However, it still is a good place to start, as without question you do need to eat better, and you most likely will need to take some quality nutritional supplements to help make up for any nutritional deficiencies.

In the beginning, a person with poor digestive problems might need to take digestive enzymes to help digest their food, as well as any nutritional supplements they take. But just as is the case when taking medication, one shouldn't have to rely on taking supplements forever for digestive purposes.

Many people can also benefit from a purification program, which can do wonders in fixing digestive issues. Of course this isn't an easy process, and so for many patients I usually will have them make small changes in the beginning. Then if and when they're ready they can begin a purification program to help restore their digestive function. I'll talk more about this briefly later in this chapter, as well as in the next chapter.

8 Tips To Help Improve Your Digestion

What I'd like to do now is discuss eight different things you can do in order to improve your digestion. Most of these you can do immediately, and while they might require some dramatic changes in your current lifestyle, I could almost guarantee you would feel much better than you currently do after incorporating some or all these changes. So let's take a look at how you can improve your digestion:

Healthy Digestion Tip #1: Cut out refined foods. This is something I'll speak about in greater detail during the next chapter, as you want to either minimize, or completely eliminate the refined foods from your diet. Being a realist, I don't expect most people to do the latter, as many health conscious doctors like myself eat some refined foods every now and then (of course some holistic doctors don't practice what they preach and eat way too many refined foods). But even if you minimize your consumption of refined foods then this will help greatly. You want to try eating as many whole foods as you can, and when possible eat organic meats, fruits, and vegetables.

Healthy Digestion Tip #2: Increase your fiber intake. Most people don't consume enough fiber, which is a big reason why many people are constipated. About 20 to 35 grams of fiber is needed per day,[9] and most people are lucky to consume half this amount with the way they eat. You can ensure sure you get enough fiber by eating plenty of fruits and vegetables, and eating foods such as seeds and nuts, as well as whole grains. You can also supplement fiber in your diet with a product like "Whole Food Fiber", which is a Standard Process product. But if you eat a sufficient amount of the foods I just mentioned then you should obtain enough fiber in your diet without needing a fiber supplement. Consuming a sufficient amount of fiber each day will help you to move your bowels daily, which as I mentioned in the past, is extremely important to healthy digestion.

Healthy Digestion Tip #3: Drink plenty of purified water. This is something else I'll also discuss in the next chapter, as you ideally want to drink at least half your weight in ounces each day of purified water. I know some people seem to have difficulty drinking enough water, as they prefer drinking coffee, soft drinks, or other beverages. Rather than trying to force yourself to drink 8 to 10 cups of water eat day, you can do what I personally do, which is in addition to the two daily "smoothies" I have which consist of two cups of water each, I have a 32 ounce bottle that I fill with purified water and I make it a goal to drink two of these bottles each day, and more on days when I exercise.

Healthy Digestion Tip #4: Correct any nutritional deficiencies. If you have any nutritional deficiencies, then these must be corrected in order to obtain optimal digestive health. Some of the more common deficiencies people with hyperthyroid conditions have are with Magnesium, Vitamin D, Selenium, Copper, Iodine, and the B Vitamins, just to name a few. There are of course other deficiencies people can have, and the best way to determine which ones you have is to consult with a qualified holistic doctor, who can recommend the appropriate testing to help you identify these common deficiencies.

Once it has been determined that you have one or more nutritional deficiencies, then you probably will need to take some nutritional supplements to correct this problem. Then once they have been corrected, if you eat a diet consisting of a variety of mostly whole foods, then for the most part you won't have to take many nutritional supplements. You still will most likely need to take some supplements, since nobody eats a perfect diet. Plus, you can't find all of these minerals in the foods you eat, although most of the nutrients and minerals you need will be in the foods you eat. Once again, it's best to consult with an expert rather than try doing this yourself.

Healthy Digestion Tip #5: Minimize your exposure to common food allergens. Two of the most common food allergens are gluten and dairy. And while it would be ideal to eliminate these from your diet completely, at the very least you want to minimize your exposure to them. This is the approach I take, as I don't completely avoid gluten and dairy, but I don't eat gluten-based foods or consume dairy on a regular basis. For those people who are following a natural treatment protocol, it's a good idea to completely avoid these foods for at least the first 30 days, and it would be even better if you can avoid them for a longer period of time. While one can test for these and other food allergens, when someone has a compromised immune system it is common to have false results. As a result it's not a bad idea for people to completely avoid gluten and dairy during the first three to six months of following a natural treatment protocol. However, I know this can be very challenging to do, and so as of writing this book I still recommend for my patients to avoid gluten and dairy for at least the first 30 days, and if they are willing to do this for a longer period of time that would be even better.

Healthy Digestion Tip #6: Take digestive enzymes. Many people have difficulty digesting the food they eat, and the ultimate goal should be to restore the health of your digestive system so that you can properly digest the food you consume. However, in the meantime, taking digestive enzymes can be beneficial. After all, if you just begin eating healthy foods and take nutritional supplements while your digestive system isn't functioning properly then there is an excellent chance you won't be able to properly digest these foods. How can you tell if you are digesting your food properly? Well, in addition to some of the symptoms you might experience (bloating, gas, etc.), you can usually tell by looking at your stool. Normal stool should be medium brown, shouldn't float, doesn't have an odor, and when having a bowel movement you shouldn't need to strain. If this doesn't describe the way your stool looks, then there is a good chance that you have some digestive issues. And if this is the case, until you get your digestive issues corrected, it's usually a good idea to take some quality digestive enzymes daily.

Healthy Digestion Tip #7: Maintain good eating habits. For example, you want to make sure you eat a healthy breakfast, don't skip meals, make sure you don't overeat, etc. Some of this might seem like common sense to you, but since many people have poor eating habits I thought it was important to briefly mention this here. So just make sure you eat every two to three hours after eating breakfast, and don't stuff yourself during any meal.

Healthy Digestion Tip #8: Consider a purification program. I was thinking about including this as the first tip, as many people can benefit from a purification program, and in many cases it's a good idea to do this right off the bat. But since I realize that many people won't do this immediately, I figured I'd first list some other things that are easier to begin with. And to be frank, if all you did was follow the first seven healthy digestive tips I have listed, you would notice a big improvement in your digestive function. But hopefully over time you will seriously consider incorporating a purification program.

So there you go! Eight things you can and should do in order to ensure a healthy digestive system. Rather than try knocking them out all at once, what I recommend is for you to incorporate one or two of these factors each week. For example, for the first week you can make a greater effort to consume more fiber, perhaps drink more water in week #2, etc. If you can make these changes all at once then that's great, but even following one or two of these tips each week will do wonders for your digestive health over time. So hopefully you realize how important it is not only to eat healthy, but to actually digest what you eat. Sure, this might sound like common sense to you, but obviously it isn't something most people think about, or else acid-stopping drugs wouldn't be such a popular item.

Does this mean I'm recommending that anyone who takes these drugs should immediately stop? Not necessarily, as you'll never see me advising anyone to stop taking any medication, as this is only a decision that you and/or your medical doctor can make on your own. My goal is just to educate you and provide you with the information you need to make an informed decision.

Chapter Summary

- Eating whole foods and taking quality nutritional supplements won't do you much good if you aren't properly digesting what you consume.
- Millions of people take acid-stopping medication, which can interfere with their ability to digest the food they eat.
- Just beginning to eat well and taking quality supplements alone after years of eating junk food usually won't be enough to fix a digestive problem. However, it still is a good place to start.
- Make sure you read the eight tips I listed in this chapter to help improve your digestive health.

For more information on these and other natural thyroid health topics, visit www.GravesDiseaseBook.com

CHAPTER 10

Hyperthyroid Diet Tips

WHEN I WAS diagnosed with Graves' Disease, proper nutrition definitely played a huge role in restoring my health back to normal. I probably don't need to inform you that different doctors will have varying opinions as to what is considered to be "healthy" with regards to one's diet. And let's be honest for a moment...nobody eats a "perfect" diet. In my opinion it's okay to be "bad" every now and then. For example, I once consulted with a patient who loved milkshakes, which as I'm sure you know isn't considered to be too healthy. This patient had about four or five milkshakes each week. And while it would be ideal for this person to completely eliminate milkshakes from their diet, having one every so often usually isn't a big deal with most people. And the same concept applies with other foods.

Of course there are exceptions. For example, someone with celiac disease probably won't be able to eat a gluten-based food "every now and then" without having a bad reaction. And there of course are people who shouldn't have a milkshake every now and then, or an occasional slice of pizza, etc. But some healthcare professionals expect every single one of their patients to avoid the consumption of all gluten-based foods, dairy products, and other foods for the rest of their life. Once again, some people do need to avoid these foods on a permanent basis, but for most people, eating these foods on an occasional basis after they have restored their health back to normal usually won't lead to any serious health issues.

Important Rules To Any Hyperthyroid Diet

In order to keep your blood sugar levels stable, there are three important rules to follow with any hyperthyroid diet. The first is to minimize or completely eliminate refined foods. The reason for this is because refined foods cause a spike in the blood sugar levels. As a result, if you eat refined foods frequently over a period of months and years, this will put a great deal of stress on your adrenal glands, as well as the pancreas. While it would be ideal to completely stop eating the refined foods, at the very least try to minimize the amount you consume.

The second rule involves eating breakfast, as while you don't necessarily need to eat a huge breakfast each morning, you should eat something within the first hour of waking up. This once again will help to keep your blood sugar levels stable, and will give you much needed energy to start the day. You want to make sure to incorporate some type of healthy protein, and avoid eating a breakfast high in carbohydrates (so no sugary cereals, pancakes, etc.).

The third and final rule is that you should eat regularly, as upon eating breakfast you should try to go no longer than a couple of hours in between meals. Once again, this will help to keep your blood sugar levels stable. And in addition to helping to minimize the amount of stress put on your adrenal glands, eating well and keeping your blood sugar levels stable can also make it easier to lose weight, although I realize that many people with hyperthyroidism or Graves' Disease have the opposite problem. When I first was diagnosed with Graves' Disease I personally was trying to gain weight, so I made sure to eat a good amount of quality protein, but still followed these same three rules. On the other hand, some people with hyperthyroid disorders do have problems losing weight due to them either consuming a lot of calories, taking antithyroid medication, or sometimes this is due to insulin resistance and/or an imbalance of the sex hormones (estrogen, progesterone, etc.).

Is Testing For Food Allergies A Good Idea?

Many holistic doctors will recommend for all of their patients to get tested for food allergies before putting them on a natural treatment protocol which involves changing their eating habits and eliminating certain types of foods. If you're thinking about getting tested for food allergies, going to a regular allergy doctor might not be the best option, as usually they will test for only IgE antibodies, which usually isn't sufficient. You might want to visit a holistic doctor and receive an ELISA/EIA panel, which also measures the IgG antibodies, and in my opinion is usually more accurate than testing for IgE antibodies.

However, as I briefly mentioned in the last chapter, one thing to keep in mind is that someone with a compromised immune system is more likely to have false results with such tests, which is one of the reasons why I typically don't recommend these food allergy panels to my patients before beginning a natural treatment protocol. If they are to receive such a test I usually advise them to receive it once they have restored their health back to normal and their immune system is healthy and strong.

Another alternative to consider is a GI Health Panel. The company Diagnos-Techs offers this type of test, which measures the health of the gastrointestinal tract and includes over one dozen tests which utilize saliva and stool specimens. They also offer a FIP-Food Intolerance Panel, which will determine whether you are allergic to four of the most common foods (gluten, soy, milk, and egg proteins). Once again, false results are common with someone who has a compromised immune system. There are other companies besides Diagnos-Techs which will perform similar tests.

A less costly approach you can take is to conduct an elimination diet, where you eliminate all of the common food allergens (wheat, soy, dairy, etc.), and then slowly introduce a potential food allergen, one at a time. There are different ways of doing this, but here is an example: You can go on a purification program (described shortly), and then once you have completed the purification program, you can introduce wheat for three days, and see how your body reacts. Just make sure you don't add more than one potential allergen at a time, as if you were to add both wheat and dairy for example, and then had a bad reaction, you wouldn't know which allergen was responsible for this. One huge downside of this approach is that people with food allergies don't always have overt symptoms when exposed to food allergens.

A Purification Program Can Be Beneficial

As I briefly mentioned in the previous chapter, many people can benefit from a purification program. There are different types of these programs, and when following one it is wise to be under the guidance of a competent healthcare professional. When I put one of my patients on a purification program, I prefer having them avoid gluten, dairy, soy, and other common food allergens for at least 21 to 30 days, and sometimes longer than this. Once again, the reason for this is because they are common allergens, and in order to restore the health of their digestive system back to normal it's a good idea to have people avoid these types of foods. Truth to be told, many people should avoid these common allergens for longer than 21 to 30 days, although for most people it's tough enough laying off such foods for one month, let alone three to six months, which in many cases would be ideal.

During a purification program I encourage my patients to eat plenty of fresh vegetables, some fruits, as well as chicken, turkey, and certain types of deep sea fish. I do recommend that they purchase organic food, at least with regards to the meats. While it would be great if they can buy everything organic, I realize some people can't afford to do this, and so if you must pick and choose, I'd recommend to eat organic meat, and try to stay away from certain non-organic vegetables and fruits which are high in pesticides. Most people can also consume a small amount of lentils and brown rice during the purification program. The 21-day purification program I recommend actually advises people not to eat any meat for the first ten days. However, I allow my patients to eat some meat, although some choose to follow the program as is and don't consume any meat until day eleven of the program.

Such a diet can obviously be a big challenge to follow for someone who is accustomed to eating junk food on a regular basis. As a result, I have some people take this slowly, as rather than immediately put them on a purification program, I will have them slowly change their eating habits until they are mentally prepared to begin such a program. This usually takes at least a few weeks, although sometimes it can take longer. Some holistic doctors recommend that every one of their patients begin such a program immediately, but in my experience I find that patient compliance is lower when you have them abruptly stop eating all junk food at once, and that people are more likely to follow through when taking this slowly. Of course some people want to begin such a program immediately, which is fine, but many people aren't ready to make such dramatic changes.

Put Together A Food Diary

Before beginning your "thyroid diet", it's also a good idea to write down everything you eat for at least one week. This not only includes the major meals you eat, but every snack, beverage, etc. This will make you more aware of what you're putting into your body, and if you're working with a natural doctor then it will also provide them with valuable information as they assist you in the process of eating healthier. After all, many of us think we're eating healthy, when in reality we're eating foods that aren't too good for us, are difficult to digest, etc.

An Actual Example Of A Hyperthyroid Diet You Can Follow:

I know you're probably eager to know what a "healthy" diet is for someone who has hyperthyroidism or Graves' Disease. So I've decided to include an example of a daily hyperthyroid diet I followed when I was first diagnosed with Graves' Disease. Keep in mind that this is just an example, and is not a diet that I stayed on permanently, (although it did train me to eat better, and I still eat healthy to this day). Plus, you of course can make modifications to this diet, and you don't need to eat the same exact foods every single day. Anyway, let's take a look at this diet:

6 am: Breakfast: Smoothie which contained two cups of purified water, one cup of mixed berries (raspberries, blueberries, and blackberries), a healthy form of protein powder (I used two scoops of SP Complete from Standard Process, which really isn't a "protein powder", but is a whole food supplement. You can substitute a healthy form of whey protein if you'd prefer), and add one teaspoon of flax oil (after one month I began adding one raw organic egg to this).

8am: Mid-morning snack #1: one serving of organic apples

10am: Mid-morning snack #2: ½ cup of raw sunflower seeds

Noon: Lunch: Grilled chicken salad: organic mixed greens and spinach, organic grilled chicken

2pm: Mid-afternoon snack #1: a Standard Process cocoa cherry bar (okay, not exactly a whole food, but definitely a healthier type of protein bar) or one serving of fresh vegetables

4pm: Mid-afternoon snack # 2: another smoothie

6pm: Dinner: Organic chicken or turkey, one or two servings of mixed vegetables

7:30pm: Snack: ½ cup of raw almonds

Although this diet is relatively healthy, you'll notice that it isn't perfect. Some people have questioned my consumption of protein bars when I initially followed a natural treatment protocol. I didn't eat protein bars every single day, as I had one daily about three or four times each week. While the ones I ate were without question healthier than most of the protein bars sold in retail stores, I probably should have substituted the protein bars with more vegetables, but overall it was a healthy diet. Today I still eat healthy, but I do incorporate some whole grains occasionally (for example, I will have a turkey wrap or sandwich with whole wheat bread), and every now and then I'll even go out and eat some pizza, chocolate, etc.

Once again, if you currently eat a lot of junk food and/or have strong sweet and carbohydrate cravings, I wouldn't expect you to change your eating habits overnight. Under such circumstances it is best to take it slow, and when I first consult with a patient who has strong sweet and carbohydrate cravings, I put them on a protocol to help them get rid of these cravings, and thus make the transition to a healthier diet much easier. I personally was brought up eating sugary cereals, plenty of fast food, and had soft drinks (punch, soda, etc.) on a daily basis. And while I was already eating much healthier when I was diagnosed with Graves' Disease, it still wasn't an easy process. But knowing that this not only can help restore your thyroid health back to normal, but will also benefit your overall health, is a huge motivator.

Drink Plenty Of Purified Water

You also want to drink plenty of purified water, avoid any soft drinks, and even most juices, which can be high in sugar. As for what type of water you should drink, different doctors have different opinions, but I recommend either water that has gone through a reverse osmosis process, or a good quality spring water. Some people will disagree with me, as some claim that water which has gone through a reverse osmosis process doesn't hydrate the body well, while others will tell you not to drink spring water, even if it is from a good source. Some will recommend distilled water, while others will tell you to drink ionized water. Of course one does need to keep in mind that drinking water from plastic bottles can expose you to xenoestrogens. So I would try to avoid drinking water from plastic bottles on a regular basis, and definitely try to stay away from tap water.

Should People With Hyperthyroidism and Graves' Disease Consume Goitrogens?

Goitrogens interfere with the function of the thyroid gland, which admittedly isn't as big of a factor in someone with a hyperthyroid condition like Graves" Disease as it would be with someone with a hypothyroid condition. However, this doesn't mean I recommend that people with hyperthyroidism and Graves' Disease should intentionally eat these foods. So even though you have a hyperthyroid condition you still want to at least minimize the following foods, and some of them you may want to avoid completely. I personally ate some of the following goitrogens in moderation (i.e. spinach and broccoli) while following a purification program, and completely avoided others (i.e. soy). Anyway, here are some of the goitrogens to be aware of:

- Soy (especially unfermented soy)
- Broccoli
- Brussels sprouts
- Cauliflower
- Kale
- Spinach
- Turnips
- Peaches
- Strawberries

Where Should You Shop?

As for where should you buy your food, although you can shop at your local health food store, I personally like Trader Joes, which is a national chain that has plenty of natural and organic food at affordable prices. Some "regular" grocery stores, and even places like Wal-Mart sell some natural and organic food as well. While my wife and I love shopping at Trader Joes for many of our items, we do buy some of our foods at local health food stores, and a few items in a "regular" supermarket.

So hopefully you now have a better idea as to which foods you should eat for your hyperthyroid condition. Truth to be told, most people should eat a healthy diet consisting of whole foods, regardless of whether or not they have a hyperthyroid condition. Doing so can actually help prevent the development of such conditions, along with incorporating other lifestyle factors, such as exercising regularly, obtaining quality sleep, and doing a good job of managing stress. But for someone with hyperthyroidism or Graves" Disease, eating well can definitely help to improve their health, and is thus extremely important.

Chapter Summary

- Different doctors will have varying opinions as to what is considered to be "healthy" with regards to one's diet.
- In order to keep your blood sugar levels stable, there are three important rules to follow with any hyperthyroid diet: 1) Minimize the amount of refined foods you eat, 2) Don't skip breakfast, 3) Eat regularly
- Many doctors test for food allergies, with the ELISA/EIA panel being popular. Another option is the GI Health Panel by Diagnos-Techs.
- Before beginning your hyperthyroid diet, I recommend for people to put together a food diary where you write down everything you eat for at least one week
- Even though goitrogens interfere with thyroid function, I don't recommend for people with hyperthyroidism to intentionally consume goitrogens as a form of treatment.

For more information on these and other natural thyroid health topics, visit www.GravesDiseaseBook.com

CHAPTER 11

Nutritional Supplements and Herbs For Hyperthyroidism & Graves' Disease

CARLY WAS TAKING a few different nutritional supplements before I consulted with her. She was taking a multi-mineral vitamin, a calcium supplement, fish oils, and she was also taking a thyroid support supplement that she had purchased online. The thyroid support supplement actually did consist of some of herbs which typically help with hyperthyroidism (Motherwort, Lemon Balm, etc.), along with some other ingredients. She had been on the thyroid support supplement for about three months, and although initially taking this supplement helped with some of her hyperthyroid symptoms, she was looking to do more than just manage her symptoms naturally.

So I put her on a natural treatment protocol, recommended some different supplements and herbs for her to take, as well as modifying certain lifestyle factors. I told her that it didn't matter where she purchased the supplements and herbs, but I warned her that she needed to make sure that they were of high quality. Just as was the case with the thyroid support supplement she had taken, she noticed a quick improvement in her hyperthyroid symptoms when following the natural treatment protocol I recommended. But this time the symptoms went away permanently, and eventually her thyroid blood levels had normalized.

For those people with hyperthyroidism and Graves' Disease looking to follow a natural treatment protocol, there are numerous nutritional supplements and herbal remedies which can help to restore their health back to normal. As you probably know by now, just taking supplements and herbs alone isn't enough to accomplish this. When I was diagnosed with Graves' Disease, nutritional supplements and herbs definitely were an important part of the recovery process. On the other hand, there were other factors which were equally important in restoring my health back to normal. So if you have skipped the other chapters in this book and directly went to this one just so you can see which supplements and/or herbs you should take, then I definitely would advise you to start reading this book from the very beginning.

As I discussed in the previous chapter, eating well is essential to any successful natural treatment protocol. Those people who continue to eat a lot of refined foods and sugars can take all of the supplements they want, and they won't be able to restore their health back to normal. This doesn't necessarily mean that you will need to eliminate junk food from your diet permanently, but you will definitely need to make some lifestyle changes if you want to not only restore your health back to normal, but also want to prevent a relapse from happening.

Nutritional Supplements and Herbs I Personally Took

The following represent the nutritional supplements and herbs I took while I was on my "natural hyperthyroid treatment protocol". Some of these I still take today on a daily basis. What's important to keep in mind is that this is just an example of what I took, and not a recommendation for anyone else with a hyperthyroid condition to take. After all, while many people can benefit from taking the same supplements, not everyone needs to take all of them. Plus, depending on what is causing your hyperthyroid condition you might need to take additional supplements and/or herbs. And as I've already mentioned, different people will also require different dosages depending on their condition.

> *NOTE: Anyone with hyperthyroidism or Graves' Disease should consult with an endocrinologist or natural endocrine doctor before taking any of the following supplements.*

1. **Bugleweed (Lycopus).** Bugleweed is a great herbal remedy for most hyperthyroid conditions, as this was perhaps the main herb that helped manage my symptoms when I first began my natural hyperthyroid treatment protocol. Just like many other people who have a hyperthyroid condition, the increased heart rate and palpitations can be scary, and Bugleweed really did help with these symptoms and allowed me to avoid taking antithyroid drugs. While many people can have their hyperthyroid symptoms managed with Bugleweed, some people who take this herb don't notice much of a difference. This is especially true for some people who have severe hyperthyroid symptoms.

2. **Motherwort (Leonurus cardiaca).** This is another great herb which can help with the hyperthyroid symptoms. Even though the Bugleweed did a great job of managing my symptoms, as my heart rate and palpitations decreased dramatically upon taking it, I still was experiencing

some palpitations after a few months. But taking both Bugleweed and Motherwort together pretty much helped to eliminate the symptoms. Obviously the entire natural treatment protocol itself helped to eliminate the symptoms, but both Bugleweed and Motherwort played a big role in providing natural symptom management.

3. **Eleuthero.** Also known as Siberian Ginseng, this herb is not just specific for those who have a hyperthyroid condition. However, for someone who has adrenal problems and deals with a lot of chronic stress (which seems to describe most people these days), taking Eleuthero daily can really be beneficial, and will make it easier to cope with the stress in your life. As I've already mentioned in this book, I believe that chronic stress was a big factor in the development of my Graves' Disease condition, and I also discussed how the Adrenal Stress Index test revealed that I had weak adrenal glands. And while modifying certain lifestyle factors plays a huge role in restoring adrenal function, receiving additional adrenal support can be very beneficial.

4. **Vitamin D.** Most people are Vitamin D deficient, and a big reason for this is because many people do everything they can to avoid the sun, which is the best source of Vitamin D. And many people who do get adequate sun exposure always put on sun block, which also blocks the absorption of Vitamin D. As a result, just about everyone needs to supplement with Vitamin D3, but before you do this it is a good idea to get tested to confirm that you are indeed deficient in Vitamin D. Vitamin D deficiency can cause a lot of problems, including a compromised immune system, which can eventually lead to the development of an autoimmune thyroid disorder, increase the likelihood of certain cancers, as well as cause many other conditions. The Vitamin D Council shows some of the different conditions that Vitamin D deficiency can lead to:

"Current research has implicated vitamin D deficiency as a major factor in the pathology of at least 17 varieties of cancer as well as heart disease, stroke, hypertension, autoimmune diseases, diabetes, depression, chronic pain, osteoarthritis, osteoporosis, muscle weakness, muscle wasting, birth defects, periodontal disease, and more."

5. **Iodine.** It is assumed by many doctors that people with a hyperthyroid disorder have an excess of iodine. The reason for this is because iodine is necessary for the formation of thyroid hormone, and since people with hyperthyroidism have an excess of thyroid hormone, it is also assumed that they have an excess of iodine. This simply isn't true, as many people with hyperthyroidism actually have an iodine deficiency. This once again can be confirmed through proper testing, as there is an iodine loading test you can take to determine if you are deficient in iodine, which will then require proper supplementation to correct this deficiency. Like Vitamin D, a deficiency in iodine can lead to many different health conditions. I'm actually going to discuss iodine in greater detail in the next chapter.

6. **Selenium.** Selenium is important for the conversion of T4 to T3, and as a result, a deficiency of selenium can lead to a thyroid disorder, although in many cases it is a hypothyroid condition which develops. However, selenium is also important when it comes to immunity, and so even if you have a hyperthyroid condition such as Graves' Disease you should make sure you are not deficient in this mineral. One study showed that taking selenium for 12 months was effective in reducing thyroid antibodies.[10] Eating one ounce of raw brazil nuts each day will give you all of the selenium you need.

7. **B vitamins.** There are many different conditions in which deficiencies of the B vitamins can lead to, and so once again, you want to make sure you avoid such a deficiency. Taking a daily whole food supplement is a

good idea, as well as eating plenty of whole foods and at the same time minimizing the amount of refined foods and sugars you consume.

8. **Magnesium.** Many people are also deficient in magnesium, which has many different roles in the body, and as a result, a deficiency in magnesium can lead to numerous different conditions. Taking supplements also can help, although eating a diet consisting of a wide variety of whole foods will greatly help, including plenty of organic vegetables and raw seeds.

9. **Omega 3 fatty acids.** More and more people are taking omega three fatty acids, but you do want to make certain of a couple of things. First of all, you want to make sure you take a high quality fatty acid, as many of the fatty acids sold in retail stores are rancid, which you can usually tell if they have a "fishy" odor upon cutting the supplement open. Second, don't take too many omega three fatty acids, as this is becoming more of a problem, and while you definitely want to avoid a deficiency, at the same time you don't want to have an excess in your system, as this can lead to other health issues.

Other Supplements And Herbs To Consider:

Lemon Balm (Melissa officinalis). This is another common herb which is used to manage the symptoms of hyperthyroidism by potentially blocking thyroid hormone activity. Some people combine Bugleweed, Motherwort, and Lemon Balm in order to help with their hyperthyroid condition. I usually will have someone start with Bugleweed, and then add the other two herbs if needed. But some herbal formulas already are premade with two or three of these herbs.

Copper. Many people with hyperthyroidism and Graves' Disease have a copper deficiency, and these people of course should supplement with copper. However, it also isn't uncommon for someone to have a copper toxicity problem, which is why someone shouldn't just be given copper randomly. As usual, proper testing is necessary to determine whether someone is deficient in copper, or has a copper toxicity problem. Copper has many different roles, as it's important for immunity, as well as the health of the thyroid and adrenal glands.

Iron. It's also common for people with hyperthyroid conditions to have an iron deficiency. Many holistic doctors overlook this as a cause of the patient's fatigue. Although compromised adrenal glands can lead to fatigue, certain deficiencies can also cause this, such as iron. Keep in mind that not all anemia is due to iron, as fatigue can also be due to a copper deficiency.

L—Carnitine. Even though I didn't take L—Carnitine when diagnosed with Graves' Disease, it does seem that this can help with the hyperthyroid symptoms by blocking thyroid hormone activity.[11]

Vitamin C. When I talk about supplementing with Vitamin C, I'm referring to whole food Vitamin C. It's important to distinguish this from the Vitamin C which is sold in most health food and other retail stores, which is ascorbic acid. This is only one component of Vitamin C, as it's the autoimmune wrapper which not only isn't as effective as the entire Vitamin C complex, but some studies show that taking ascorbic acid, as well as other antioxidants, can be harmful to your health.[12]

Lithium. Some sources suggest that a deficiency in lithium can be linked to hyperthyroidism. According to the website www.ithyroid.com (which is a very interesting website that anyone with hyperthyroidism or Graves' Disease should check out), "A deficiency of lithium may cause the mineral and amino acid deficiencies seen in hyperthyroidism".

Glutathione. The same website (www.ithyroid.com) talks about how glutathione combines with Vitamin E and Selenium to form glutathione peroxidase, which helps to protect the thyroid gland from oxidation damage. I personally don't include Lithium or Glutathione as part of my natural treatment protocol for people with hyperthyroidism and Graves' Disease, and I also didn't take either of these when restoring my health back to normal. But this doesn't mean that they can't benefit people with hyperthyroid conditions.

There are other supplements and herbs which can benefit people with hyperthyroidism and Graves' Disease. For example, it's also a good idea to take a whole food multivitamin to help provide many of the necessary vitamins. Some people need to take certain supplements or herbs for digestive support. The goal here isn't to list every single nutritional supplement and herb which can benefit people with hyperthyroid conditions, but I did try to list the most important ones.

So how can you determine which of these supplements you need to take as part of a natural treatment protocol? Most people with hyperthyroidism and Graves' Disease would simply begin taking these supplements and herbs on their own, which might help a little bit, but chances are you won't receive optimal results. For example, there have been some people with a hyperthyroid condition who have taken Bugleweed on their own, only to see the Free T3 and T4 levels increase. If this happens then it's usually not due to the Bugleweed itself, but other factors. The problem is that the body is very complex, so while some people will take a combination of these supplements and herbs and then feel better without addressing the other factors I've discussed in this book, many people won't experience positive results taking this approach. Plus, even those people who do feel better usually won't restore their health back to normal just by eating well and taking some of these supplements and herbs.

This is yet another reason why it's wise to consult with a competent natural endocrine doctor, as they will evaluate your condition and put you on an individual plan depending on which nutritional deficiencies you may have, whether you have any hormonal imbalances, etc. Not only that, but they will also monitor your condition so that you're not taking these supplements longer than you need to. As I mentioned earlier, some of these supplements can and should be taken regularly (Vitamin D, fatty acids, etc.), but others do not need to be taken long-term. So rather than taking these supplements and herbs on your own, do yourself a favor and consult with a holistic doctor who focuses on endocrine disorders.

Chapter Summary

- For those people with hyperthyroidism and Graves' Disease looking to follow a natural treatment protocol, there are numerous nutritional supplements and herbal remedies which can help to restore their health back to normal.
- Those who continue to eat a lot of refined foods and sugars can take all of the supplements they want, and they still won't be able to restore their health back to normal.
- The following are some of the nutritional supplements and herbs I took when I was diagnosed with hyperthyroidism and Graves' Disease: 1) Bugleweed, 2) Motherwort, 3) Eleuthero, 4) Vitamin D, 5) Iodine, 6) Selenium, 7) B Vitamins, 8) Magnesium, 9) Omega 3 Fatty Acids

For more information on these and other natural thyroid health topics, visit www.GravesDiseaseBook.com

CHAPTER 12

The Truth About Iodine And Hyperthyroidism

MANY PEOPLE WITH hyperthyroid conditions are told to avoid iodine. Not only are they usually advised not to take any iodine supplements, but many are told to avoid foods which contain a lot of iodine, such as certain kinds of seafood. The reason for this is because many doctors assume that people with an overactive thyroid have an excessive amount of iodine. The reason for this is because iodine is essential for the production of thyroid hormone, and so if the thyroid gland is producing an excessive amount of thyroid hormone, as is the case with hyperthyroidism and Graves' Disease, then it's easy for someone to assume that there is also an excess amount of iodine.

When I was diagnosed with Graves' Disease I initially thought the same thing, as a lot of sources informed people with hyperthyroidism and Graves' Disease to avoid iodine. But after consulting with multiple holistic doctors, and doing some research of my own, I realized that many people with hyperthyroid conditions are actually deficient in iodine. Not everyone of course, but I personally was iodine deficient, and so I followed an iodine supplement protocol, which I'll talk about shortly.

How Can You Detect an Iodine Deficiency?

I'd like to discuss a couple of different methods to determine whether someone has an iodine deficiency. The first, and perhaps the least reliable method is through an Iodine Patch test. This test involves taking a 2% tincture of iodine, and essentially drawing a 2 x 2 "patch" on your forearm, stomach, or inner thigh with the iodine tincture. If a person has a sufficient amount of iodine in their body, then the patch shouldn't begin to fade significantly until after 24 hours. If it fades in less than 24 hours then the person is said to have an iodine deficiency. If it fades in 12 hours or less then the person has a more severe iodine deficiency. As you might have guessed, this isn't the most accurate way of detecting an iodine deficiency, although I do think it does have some value, especially for giving a general idea as to whether someone has an iodine deficiency.

A more accurate method of determining whether someone has an iodine deficiency is through an iodine loading test. This is a urine test which measures the amount of iodine excreted over a 24-hour period. It involves taking a 50mg tablet of iodine/iodide, and then seeing how much is excreted through the urine over the next 24 hours. It's not the most convenient test, as you need to collect ALL of your urine within a 24 hour period, as just missing a single urine sample will make the results inaccurate. If 90% of the ingested iodine/iodide is excreted, then the person has a sufficient amount of iodine. On the other hand, if they excrete less than 90% of iodine/iodide then they have an iodine deficiency.[13] So for example, a person who excretes only 20% of the iodine/iodide ingested is more iodine deficient than someone who excretes 50% of the iodine/iodide.

Keys To Beginning An Iodine Supplementation Protocol

When beginning to supplement with iodine, it's important to understand that this should be a slow process. I once visited a blog where a person was talking about using the Iodine Patch Test to determine whether or not he was iodine deficient. I like the Iodine Patch Test, but as I briefly mentioned before, it's definitely not the most accurate test. In any case, the "blogger" used the iodine patch test to determine that he was iodine deficient, and then he ingested a large amount of iodine daily for about two weeks, and then did a follow up iodine patch test. When re-testing after two weeks he didn't notice any significant difference with regards to how long it took for the iodine patch to disappear.

However, one thing he didn't realize is that you can't force your body to "make up" for an iodine deficiency in two weeks by ingesting large amounts of iodine. It's not that easy, as it usually takes months to correct such a deficiency. I followed the protocol recommended by Dr. Janet Lang, and the same protocol is also recommended by Donna Wild, who has more than 20 years of experience using whole food nutritional concentrates, and has an excellent presentation about the benefits of iodine. Based on this advice I personally began by taking a 3 mg tablet of an iodine supplement called Prolamine Iodine daily for one week, and then added an additional 3 mg tablet each week until I was taking 24 mg.

You might wonder how much iodine you specifically need to correct your deficiency (assuming you have one of course). According to "iodine expert" Dr. David Brownstein, you can take up to 50 mg of iodine per day, and even higher than this if you have an extremely severe deficiency.[4] As for how much iodine YOU specifically will need to take, this is something that will be determined through the initial test results and then through follow-up testing, which is yet another good reason to consult with a competent holistic doctor.

Why People With Hashimoto's Thyroiditis Need To Be Careful About Taking Iodine

People with Hashimoto's Thyroiditis need to avoid taking iodine until the autoimmune response has been addressed. If they take iodine while their thyroid antibodies are still high, their symptoms most likely will worsen. Once the immune system component has been addressed, the person can then begin an iodine loading protocol if they are deficient in iodine. However, in my experience, most people with Graves' Disease who have an iodine deficiency usually don't need to have the autoimmune response addressed before they can begin such a protocol.

Research Studies Show That Iodine Can Help With Hyperthyroidism and Graves' Disease

While some people recommend that all people with hyperthyroid conditions should avoid iodine, certain research studies show that taking iodine can help with hyperthyroidism and Graves' Disease. Once again, the person should be tested first to confirm an iodine deficiency. And one really should be under the guidance of a competent holistic doctor before beginning a supplementation program. One study with the Danish population involving 8,219 looked at the effect of higher iodine intake on thyroid hormone, and discovered that consuming higher amounts of iodine led to a lower prevalence of hyperthyroidism.[15] Another study showed that patients with hyperthyroidism given 2mg or 4mg of iodine daily showed thyroid inhibition, and that "improvement was apparent within 48 hours".[16]

Once again, I'm proof that someone with a hyperthyroid condition can take iodine without a problem. And many of my patients with hyperthyroidism and Graves' Disease take iodine as well. Of course I don't just randomly give high dosages of iodine to all of my patients, as I always recommend testing for a deficiency first. And when someone is deficient I always start them out with a low dosage of iodine.

Dr. David Brownstein has written a book called, "Iodine, Why You Need It, Why You Can't Live Without It". Even though this might sound like a boring book to read, it actually is very interesting, plus it's an easy-to-read book. In any case, Dr. Brownstein has done a lot of research involving iodine, and has determined that most people are iodine deficient. In fact, in his book he states the following: "The rising incidence of Hashimoto's and Graves' Disease correlates with falling iodine levels. I believe the increase in both Hashimoto's and Graves' Disease is due in large part to iodine deficiency."[17] I promise that after reading this book you'll be amazed at how important iodine is, and will also learn why most people are deficient in it.

Chapter Summary

- Although many "experts" advise people with hyperthyroidism to avoid iodine, many people with hyperthyroidism and Graves' Disease have an iodine deficiency.
- Two methods to determine whether someone has an iodine deficiency are 1) the iodine patch test, and 2) the iodine loading test
- When beginning to supplement with iodine, it's important to understand that this should be a slow process.
- I highly recommend reading the book "Iodine, Why You Need It, Why You Can't Live Without It", which was written by Dr. David Brownstein.

For more information on these and other natural thyroid health topics, visit www.GravesDiseaseBook.com

CHAPTER 13

Can Environmental Toxins Trigger Graves' Disease?

THERE IS A book called the Autoimmune Epidemic, which talks about how autoimmune conditions are on the rise, yet they still don't gain the attention that cancer and heart disease have received. The author talks a great deal about how environmental toxins are potentially responsible for many of the autoimmune conditions which exist.

There are over one hundred autoimmune conditions, and the bad news is that someone with Graves' Disease or Hashimoto's Thyroiditis seems more likely to develop one or more additional autoimmune conditions when compared to the general public. This makes sense when you think about it, as someone with a compromised immune system will be more susceptible to other autoimmune disorders, as I mentioned in an earlier chapter.

Although I talk a great deal about how lifestyle factors and nutritional deficiencies can contribute to or directly cause an autoimmune thyroid disorder, one can't discount the impact toxins have. After all, in this day and age we are being exposed to toxins which weren't as prominent decades ago. And so perhaps it is of no coincidence that as we are being exposed to more environmental toxins, the rate of autoimmune conditions is increasing. As Donna Jackson Nakazawa reveals in the book the Autoimmune Epidemic, companies aren't required to report whether these toxins can do harm to the immune system:

"While chemical companies have to divulge information if their chemicals have been found to be carcinogenic in lab testing, no such testing and reporting are required on whether chemicals act as autogens and damage the human immune system".[18]

Being Careful About What You Bring Into Your Home

The bad news is that unlike lifestyle factors, you don't have complete control with regards to the toxins you're exposed to on a daily basis. It is impossible to avoid all of the environmental toxins out there, but most people can do a better job of minimizing their exposure to them. A big area is with the household products people buy, as this is a huge problem which exposes people to many of these toxins.

One of the primary toxins we're exposed to on a frequent basis is xenohormones. And when trying to restore one's health through a natural treatment protocol, xenohormones are one of the main factors which can affect a person's recovery. While many people with thyroid conditions are aware they need to eat better, exercise more, and modify other lifestyle factors, most people don't pay enough attention to xenohormones. So what I'd like to do is briefly talk about what xenohormones are, how they affect your health, and what you can do to minimize your exposure to them.

Xenohormones are substances which contain synthetic hormones, primarily estrogen, and therefore have a hormone-like effect on the body. Many of today's products and foods contain synthetic hormones, which without question have a profound effect on our endocrine systems, as well as our overall health. Some of the products and foods which contain xenohormones include:

- Pesticides
- Herbicides
- Fungicides
- Detergents
- Nail polish and nail polish remover
- Meat from livestock fed hormones to increase their size
- Many non-organic dairy products
- Many cosmetics
- Paint remover
- Some types of soaps
- Glues
- Most plastics (so be careful about drinking too much bottled water)
- Many perfumes and air fresheners

While xenohormones can affect the health of anyone with a thyroid condition (as well as those people who don't have a thyroid disorder), people with an autoimmune thyroid disorder are arguably affected even more. So those people with Graves' Disease and Hashimoto's Thyroiditis need to take extra precautions in order to minimize their exposure to xenohormones, as they can have a negative effect on the immune system.

In fact, here is a quote from the book entitled "What Your Doctor May Not Tell You About Menopause", which was written by Dr. John R. Lee:

"More recent research is showing that exposure to xenohormones suppresses the immune-system, and in particular hampers T-lymphocyte

function, and lowers the proportions and numbers of natural killer (NK) cells. These are two of your immune system's most important defenses. The latest studies are showing even more widespread damage to the immune system." [19]

In addition to weakening one's immune system, there are many other side effects that xenohormones can have. Keep in mind that most of the time the effects aren't immediate, as it takes years for these symptoms and conditions to develop. But some of the different symptoms include fatigue, headaches, depression, lack of concentration, increased mood swings and irritability, and many other symptoms.

If this sounds similar to some of the side effects of a hormone imbalance, this is because xenohormones essentially disrupt the endocrine system, and therefore create a hormone imbalance. The reason for this is because they closely resemble our natural hormones, which allows them to bind to the same receptors. So for example, synthetic estrogens will bind to the estrogen receptors. But they don't have the same functions as natural estrogens, which is why they will cause many different side effects.

But they cause more than just side effects. As mentioned previously, exposure to these toxins can potentially lead to the development of an autoimmune condition. Research studies also show that long-term exposure to xenohormones can also increase the incidence of certain types of cancers. So hopefully you're beginning to realize how dangerous these toxins are, and will begin trying to do everything you can to minimize your exposure to them.

And if you are of childbearing age and are thinking of having children, keep in mind that studies also show that xenohormones can affect future generations.[20] So when a patient of mine informs me that she is trying to get pregnant, one of the things I'll recommend is for her to begin a purification program to help clean out some of the toxins, including many of these xenohormones. This will help to put her in a better state of health before she becomes pregnant and help to minimize her babies' exposure to these toxins.

It is of course impossible to avoid all of the environmental toxins out there. However, as I have already mentioned, many of the xenohormones we're exposed to are a result of the foods and products we bring into our own homes, and so this is something we CAN control. One of the problems is that currently companies don't need to reveal whether or not they include synthetic hormones in their foods and products, although this may soon change. As a result, your best bet is to try to purchase as many organic foods and products as possible, and if you buy non-organic products, use brands which don't have xenohormones.

There are numerous books that discuss the problems involved with xenohormones. But if you don't want to read an entire book, simply taking 30 minutes to read the "Xenobiotics chapter" in the book I mentioned before (What Your Doctor May Not Tell You About Menopause) will really help you to better understand the consequences of these toxins.

When you think about it, there is really no good reason to purchase all of these products which contain potentially harmful chemicals and toxins. Especially when there are natural alternatives out there for most of these products. Sure, they will most likely cost more than the brand-name products most people buy, but it's definitely worth the extra money spent.

Can Air Fresheners Cause Asthma?

Plus, some of these chemicals shouldn't be used at all in my opinion. For example, I remember when growing up as a child my mother constantly would use air fresheners in our house. Just like most people, she didn't realize the potential damage these chemicals can cause to the lungs and other tissues in the body when used frequently. Perhaps it's no coincidence that she eventually developed asthma (although to be fair, she did smoke for many years as well, which obviously can be a big factor). I'm not suggesting that everyone who uses air fresheners will develop asthma, or any other health condition for that matter. However, many people use similar chemicals, and assume that they are completely safe, but many of them aren't.

The book "The Autoimmune Epidemic" goes beyond household products, and it's definitely a book that's worth reading. The reason why I'm spending a lot of time focusing on household products is because this is a big area in which most people can control. But the book discussed other ways in which we're commonly exposed to toxins. It even briefly spoke about some of the dangers of the toxins present in vaccines, which obviously is a very controversial topic and is not something I really want to get into in this book.

The overall point of this chapter was to make you aware that there are many things in our environment we don't think of as being toxic. I guarantee that most women don't put on nail polish realizing that this is a toxin. And of course many parents put nail polish on their children's fingernails as well. Another thing to keep in mind is that some of these "toxins" might take years to cause the development of an autoimmune condition, although some people might never develop any condition from exposure to these toxins. In fact, I think it's safe to say that most women won't develop Graves' Disease just because they use nail polish.

On the other hand, the combination of nail polish and other toxic cosmetics, household cleaners, and other products may very well increase their chances of developing Graves' Disease or another autoimmune condition. The truth is we don't completely know the impact of these chemicals on our health, but as I mentioned before, since there are alternative options out there it makes sense to purchase products that are natural and try everything you can to avoid chemicals which can potentially trigger an autoimmune response.

In summary, the number of environmental toxins we've been exposed to over the years have increased dramatically, as has the number of autoimmune thyroid conditions such as Graves' Disease. And while some might dismiss this as being a coincidence, books like "The Autoimmune Epidemic", as well as others, show that environmental toxins probably do play a role in the increased incidence of these conditions. So hopefully this chapter motivates you to begin purchasing more natural products and foods, which will help greatly in minimizing your exposure to these toxins.

Chapter Summary

- Although in this book I talk a great deal about how lifestyle factors and nutritional deficiencies can contribute to or directly cause an autoimmune thyroid disorder, one can't discount the impact environmental toxins have.

- It is impossible to avoid all of the environmental toxins out there, but most people can do a better job of minimizing their exposure to them. Many of the toxins we're exposed to are cosmetics and other household products we buy.

- One of the primary toxins we're exposed to is xenohormones. Xenohormones are substances which contain synthetic hormones, primarily estrogen, and therefore have a hormone-like effect on the body.

- While xenohormones can affect the health of anyone with a thyroid condition (as well as those people who don't have a thyroid disorder), people with an autoimmune thyroid disorder are arguably affected even more.

For more information on these and other natural thyroid health topics, visit www.GravesDiseaseBook.com

CHAPTER 14

How Big Of A Role Does Genetics Play?

I'M SURE MANY people with hyperthyroidism and Graves' Disease wonder whether genetics play a major role in the development of their disorder. In fact, I've had numerous patients ask me as to whether genetics is the primary reason why they have developed a hyperthyroid or autoimmune thyroid condition, and whether this would prevent them from receiving good results when following a natural treatment protocol.

The truth is that many people with thyroid conditions have genetic markers which will make them more susceptible to developing such a condition. However, research is showing that just because someone has a genetic marker for a thyroid or autoimmune thyroid condition does not necessarily mean they will develop such a disorder. Although genetics does play a role, more and more studies are showing that lifestyle and environmental factors play an even greater role. In fact, thyroid health expert Mary J Shomon reveals the following on the website www.thy-roid-info.com regarding genetics and autoimmune disease:

> *"Genetic factors can affect an individual's immune system and its responses to foreign antigens in several ways. Genes determine the variety of MHC molecules that individuals carry on their cells. Genes also influence the potential array of T-cell receptors present on T cells. In fact, some MHC genes are associated with autoimmune diseases. However, genes are not the only factors involved in determining a person's susceptibility to an autoimmune disease. For example, some individuals who carry disease-associated MHC molecules on their cells will not develop an autoimmune disease."* [21]

The author of The Autoimmune Epidemic also reveals the following:

> *"Twin studies show that autoimmune disease is roughly 30 percent genetic and 70 percent environmental. While two identical twins might hold the same genetic code for a certain autoimmune disease, either one of them will be struck with disease only if they meet up with the right environmental hit. As one researcher put it, while genetics may load the gun, it's environment that pulls the trigger."* [22]

So even if you happen to have a genetic marker specifically for Graves' Disease, this does not mean you will develop this condition. And if you already have Graves' Disease, you can still restore your health back to normal by following a natural treatment protocol, even if you do have a genetic marker.

This obviously is good news, as while some people might have an increased chance of developing hyperthyroidism or Graves' Disease due to genetic factors, most of these people who don't have a such a condition can take steps to prevent such a disorder from developing. And as I've already mentioned, those people who do have an existing hyperthyroid condition can potentially restore their health back to normal by following a natural treatment protocol, despite having a genetic marker for such a disorder.

Other Resources Show That Lifestyle Factors Play An Important Role

Obviously I don't expect anyone to simply take my word for it that lifestyle factors play an equally important role, and perhaps an even greater role than genetics in determining whether or not someone develops a thyroid or autoimmune thyroid condition. I've already listed some resources which show that this is true. But if you want to read more about this, there are a few books out there that will discuss the importance of lifestyle factors when it comes to developing certain conditions. One book is called "Outsmart Your Genes: How Understanding Your DNA Will Empower You to Protect Yourself Against Cancer, Alzheimer's, Heart Disease, Obesity, and Many Other Conditions", which is written Dr. Scott Colby, and he goes into detail about genetics and predictive medicine, and how using genetic testing can help prevent the development of certain conditions, including thyroid disorders. Another book, called the "Biology of Belief", by Bruce Lipton, also talks about genetics and how genes and DNA aren't the sole factors when it comes to developing certain conditions.

Just keep in mind that these books aren't specific to thyroid conditions. For example, in the book "Outsmart Your Genes", Dr. Colby talks about some of the different conditions which are determined by a combination of genetic and nongenetic factors. In addition to thyroid conditions, other examples of such conditions include heart disease, cancer, Parkinson's, Alzheimer's, and arthritis. Without question, there are certain diseases which are solely determined by genetics, and aren't influenced by lifestyle factors. Some examples include Tay-Sachs Disease and cystic fibrosis. While there might not be much we can do to prevent or cure a disease such as cystic fibrosis, many of these other conditions can be prevented or in some cases completely cured.

How To Find Out If You Have A Genetic Marker For A Thyroid Condition

These days it is actually possible to find out if you have a genetic marker for a thyroid condition, along with other conditions. I'm not going to go into detail about this, as if you read the book "Outsmart Your Genes", it will talk about how you can find out which genetic markers you have through genetic testing. In his book Dr. Colby also includes examples of labs where you can go to obtain such testing.

While I think this information can be useful, I'm definitely not at the point where I would recommend that my patients receive genetic testing to find out if they have a genetic marker for a thyroid condition. Because in all honesty it's not going to change my approach with regards to the natural treatment protocol I'm going to recommend. One advantage such testing could have is that it would make people more aware of the conditions they are susceptible to. So perhaps people would be more compliant with following a natural treatment protocol if they knew they had a genetic marker for a thyroid condition. In any case, I of course don't require, or even bring up genetic testing when consulting with patients, and I don't see this changing in the near future.

Will Having A Genetic Marker Prevent Hyperthyroidism or Graves' Disease From Being Permanently Cured?

As I have already mentioned numerous times, people with a genetic marker for a hyperthyroid condition can restore their health through natural treatment methods. However, you might wonder if having a marker would prevent your condition from being permanently cured. In other words, even if following a natural treatment protocol restores your health back to normal, will having this genetic marker put you at risk of having a relapse in the future? I don't know if there is a specific answer to this, but my response is "probably so". The reason is because while a natural treatment protocol can potentially restore the health of someone with a hyperthyroid condition, if someone has a genetic marker for this condition, and then goes on to neglect those lifestyle factors I have discussed in this book, then there is a good chance they will suffer a relapse over time.

However, this might also hold true for those people who don't have a genetic marker for a thyroid condition. In other words, if someone without a genetic marker develops a thyroid condition solely due to lifestyle factors, restores their health through natural treatment methods, and then neglects their health again, then there is a good chance they will suffer a relapse.

This is yet another reason why I don't like to use the word "cure", as my goal is not to cure any condition, but rather is to help the person achieve optimal health and then show them how to maintain their health. I of course spoke about this in detail in a previous chapter, talking about the difference between a permanent cure and a state of remission. And as I've already mentioned, I don't know if someone without a genetic marker can be considered to be permanently cured, let alone someone who does have a genetic marker. Either way, one needs to maintain their health or there is a chance their condition can return.

So while there is always a chance for a relapse to occur whether someone has a genetic marker or not, if you do restore your health back to normal and then maintain your health, then this will obviously decrease the chances of you suffering a relapse. In summary, genetics is without question a factor when developing a thyroid condition, but it isn't the only factor. Lifestyle factors at least play an equally important role, and these factors may actually be more important than genetics.

Chapter Summary

- Research is showing that just because someone has a genetic marker for a thyroid or autoimmune thyroid condition does not necessarily mean they will develop such a disorder.
- These days it is actually possible to find out if you have a genetic marker for a thyroid condition, along with other conditions.
- Lifestyle factors can play a greater role in determining whether someone will develop a thyroid or autoimmune thyroid disorder.

For more information on these and other natural thyroid health topics, visit www.GravesDiseaseBook.com

CHAPTER 15

Graves' Disease & Thyroid Antibodies

IF SOMEONE HAS positive TSI antibodies then they have Graves' Disease. This is true even if other thyroid blood tests are negative, as it's important to understand that in most cases, the autoimmune response will develop first, and will usually be followed by malfunctioning of the thyroid gland.

This might seem to be confusing to those people with Graves' Disease who consider their condition to be a thyroid disorder. Even though I and other healthcare professionals refer to Graves' Disease as an autoimmune thyroid disorder, it really is an autoimmune condition which leads to thyroid malfunction. In other words, the malfunctioning thyroid gland is usually not the actual cause of the disorder in an autoimmune thyroid condition, as I have already discussed in other chapters.

So while most people with Graves' Disease have a low TSH and/or a high free T4, one can be positive for thyroid antibodies without having these other blood tests positive. How does this process develop? Elaine Moore does a wonderful job discussing the different types of antibodies in her book "Graves Disease, A Practical Guide". She discusses how the "TSI acts as an agonist, mimicking TSH and causing excess thyroid hormone production".[23] So this antibody will cause an excess of thyroid hormone, which eventually will lead to the low TSH and high free T3 and T4 levels. She also discusses the thyroid growth stimulating immunoglobulins (TGI), and states that "when Graves' Disease patients are tested for both TGI and TSI, nearly 100 percent of patients are positive for one or the other antibody".[24]

Many people with Graves' Disease also have positive TPO antibodies. These confirm the presence of an autoimmune thyroid condition, but they aren't specific to Graves' Disease, as most people with Hashimoto's Thyroiditis will also have positive TPO antibodies. Regardless of the type of thyroid antibodies you have, the obvious goal will be to restore the health of your immune system so that all of these levels will be negative.

What Determines Which Autoimmune Thyroid Condition One Will Develop?

Why do some people develop Graves' Disease, while other people develop Hashimoto's Thyroiditis? It's a matter of having different antibodies, as different antibodies will act on different parts of the thyroid gland. Genetics of course is a factor as to which thyroid antibodies a person will develop. The truth is that there is still a lot we don't know about why someone develops a specific autoimmune condition such as Graves' Disease instead of Hashimoto's Thyroiditis, or vice versa.

While I'm sure in the future we will discover even more about autoimmune thyroid conditions, what's important to understand for now is that in order to restore the health of anyone who has an autoimmune condition, one needs to do more than manage the symptoms. This is where conventional medicine fails, as most conventional medical treatments are aimed at managing the symptoms of the autoimmune condition, as you have learned in this book. This isn't just the case with Graves' Disease, but with many other autoimmune conditions as well. For example, someone with Hashimoto's Thyroiditis will almost always be told to take synthetic or natural thyroid hormone, but nothing will be done to address the autoimmune response. So the person will take thyroid hormone daily to help with the symptoms while their thyroid gland continues to be damaged by the thyroid antibodies.

It's a similar situation with Graves' Disease, as when I was initially diagnosed by my endocrinologist, she recommended antithyroid drugs, along with a beta blocker to manage my symptoms. And while she didn't really talk much about radioactive iodine treatment, there is little doubt that if I decided to take the antithyroid drugs and if they failed to put my condition into remission, then RAI probably would have been brought up as the "solution". But nothing was ever mentioned by her as to how I should restore the health of my immune system, adrenal glands, and other compromised areas of my body, and this is how most endocrinologists and other types of medical doctors think. Most don't try to do anything to cure the condition, but are trained to simply manage the symptoms.

Thyroid Antibodies Test Won't Always Be Positive

It's also important to know that someone with an autoimmune thyroid condition such as Graves' Disease won't always have positive thyroid antibodies. So if you had a thyroid antibodies test and it came out negative, this doesn't mean that you don't have an autoimmune condition. This is why it's important to also consider the patient's symptoms, other thyroid blood tests (although once again these might be negative as well), along with other factors.

Because of this, if someone with Graves' Disease follows a natural treatment protocol, how do they know if they have been cured? In other words, if they initially had positive thyroid antibodies, but after a few months of following a natural treatment protocol they have a negative test, how can one be sure if their health has been restored back to normal? The answer is that you can't confirm that someone has had their health restored just by looking at the levels of thyroid antibodies. You need to look at many different factors, including their thyroid blood test results, other tests that might be recommended (ASI test, hormone panel, hair mineral analysis, etc.), and of course their symptoms.

So based on what I've discussed so far, how does someone who is diagnosed with hyperthyroidism but has tested negative for thyroid antibodies know for sure they don't have Graves' Disease? According to some medical doctors this can confirmed through a radioactive iodine uptake test, which I'm about to discuss.

What You Need To Know About The Radioactive Iodine Uptake Test

Many people with hyperthyroidism receive a test called the Radioactive Iodine Uptake test. With this test the patient swallows a small dosage of radioactive iodine. Since the thyroid gland uses iodine to produce thyroid hormone, it will absorb the small dosage of radioactive iodine. The absorption of the radioactive iodine is evaluated after six hours, and then again after 24 hours.

If the uptake of radioiodine is high then this indicates that your thyroid gland is producing an excess of thyroxine. This is usually due to Graves' Disease, but can also be related to thyroid nodules. If your radioiodine uptake test is low, but it's confirmed that you have hyperthyroidism, then you probably have thyroiditis. So the radioactive iodine uptake test doesn't really offer 100% confirmation that someone has Graves' Disease, although this test can give the medical doctor a better idea as to whether a person has this condition.

Will The Radioactive Iodine Uptake Test Damage Your Thyroid Gland?

I have received some emails from people who didn't want to receive this test because they were afraid it would damage their thyroid gland. Part of this is probably due to the fact that I frequently talk about the risks of radioactive iodine treatment, and how one should avoid this treatment method if at all possible.

But it's important to understand that the dosage given for the radioactive iodine uptake test is much smaller than the dosage given during radioactive iodine treatment. So does this mean that it's completely harmless to the thyroid gland? Well, any procedure which involves radiation isn't completely harmless, even if the dosage is small. But this test most likely won't destroy enough thyroid cells to have a significant impact on thyroid function.

So should everyone with hyperthyroidism receive the radioactive iodine uptake test in order to rule out Graves' Disease? I wouldn't necessarily recommend this, as if someone tests positive for hyperthyroidism and also has a positive test for thyroid antibodies, then in my opinion it's usually not necessary to receive this test. On the other hand, if the thyroid antibodies test is negative, then obtaining the radioactive iodine uptake test can possibly help to determine if someone has Graves' Disease.

After all, just because someone has a negative test for thyroid antibodies doesn't mean they don't have Graves' Disease, as I have already discussed. And so if someone has a negative reading for thyroid antibodies then it might be a good idea to receive the radioactive iodine uptake test. On the other hand, for someone who is looking to receive conventional medical treatment, receiving this test probably won't make much of a difference with regards to the treatment protocol. Chances are you will be told to take antithyroid drugs or receive RAI regardless of whether you have a positive or negative radioactive iodine uptake test. And this isn't just based on my opinion, as some studies suggest that the radioactive iodine uptake test doesn't really do much when it comes to predicting the outcome of certain conventional treatment methods, such as RAI.[25] Although it can determine if someone has thyroid nodules, this can usually be determined through an ultrasound, which is less invasive than a radioactive iodine uptake test.

The same concept applies with someone who wants to follow a natural treatment protocol. Most holistic doctors aren't going to just rely on the conventional medical tests when devising a treatment plan. So for most people, receiving a radioactive iodine uptake test won't have much of an impact as to what type of treatment they would receive.

Contraindications Of This Test

Women who are pregnant or breastfeeding shouldn't receive this test.[26] The reason is because while the small dosage of iodine isn't enough to cause harm to an adult, it can cause problems with a fetus or baby. If you're not sure whether or not you are pregnant, but suspect you might be, then it's best to hold off on this test.

To summarize this chapter, the presence of thyroid antibodies is confirmation for an autoimmune thyroid condition. TSI antibodies specifically confirm the presence of Graves' Disease. On the other hand, a negative test for thyroid antibodies doesn't mean that someone doesn't have Graves' Disease. For someone with positive antibodies, it shouldn't come to a surprise that following a natural treatment protocol may result in future negative tests for thyroid antibodies. Even though one can't rely on the presence or absence of these levels, it still is a good feeling when someone has had multiple tests for thyroid antibodies, all of which were positive, and then to see these same tests come out negative after following a natural treatment protocol.

As for the radioactive iodine uptake test, although this treatment method won't obliterate the thyroid gland, it still does involve a small dosage of radiation. As a result, while receiving this test shouldn't cause much harm to the thyroid gland, because it does involve some radiation I wouldn't recommend that everyone with hyperthyroidism receive it. The question you need to ask yourself is "will receiving this test affect the course of treatment?" If the answer is "yes", then it might be worth it to receive this test. On the other hand, if the answer is "no", which usually is the case, then it's probably best not to receive this test.

Chapter Summary

- If you have been tested for thyroid antibodies and the test came out positive, and if you are experiencing hyperthyroid symptoms, then this most likely means that you have Graves' Disease.
- It's important to know that someone with an autoimmune thyroid condition won't always test positive for thyroid antibodies.
- Although the Radioactive Iodine Uptake test probably won't cause permanent damage to your thyroid gland, this doesn't mean I recommend that everyone with hyperthyroidism should receive this test.
- Women who are pregnant or breastfeeding shouldn't receive the Radioactive Iodine Uptake Test.

For more information on these and other natural thyroid health topics, visit www.GravesDiseaseBook.com

CHAPTER 16

Why Radioactive Iodine Should Usually Be The Last Resort

WHEN JIM WAS diagnosed with Graves' Disease, two different endocrinologists recommended that he receive radioactive iodine treatment. Although he had moderate hyperthyroid symptoms, they were being controlled by the antithyroid drugs he was taking. Even before he stumbled upon my website he was opposed to having his thyroid gland obliterated, and so he continued taking PTU to help manage his hyperthyroid symptoms. Like many people who consult with me for the first time, Jim was very skeptical of natural treatment methods. However, he didn't want to take the antithyroid drugs for a prolonged period of time, and he wanted to do everything he could to avoid RAI.

So he eventually began a natural treatment protocol. He experienced a quick improvement in his symptoms, although there wasn't much of a change in his thyroid blood tests after he retested for the first time (after two months had gone by). I told him not to become discouraged, as everyone is different, and it was great that he was experiencing positive changes in his symptoms. He stuck with the program, saw an improvement in his blood test results two months later, and the next time he had retested (two months later) the blood tests had normalized. While many people in Jim's situation would have followed the advice of their endocrinologist and received the radioactive iodine, Jim realized that radioactive iodine should be the last resort in most cases.

In the United States, radioactive iodine is commonly recommended as the first line of treatment for people with hyperthyroidism and Graves' Disease. Sometimes this happens even when the person's hyperthyroid symptoms are mild. I have personally consulted with people with mild hyperthyroid symptoms who had their thyroid gland obliterated through radioactive iodine. Many endocrinologists will recommend RAI based on the thyroid blood tests alone. In other words, if someone has a low TSH and/or high free T4 levels, they will recommend radioactive iodine to that patient, regardless of how mild their symptoms might be.

The following represent three reasons why radioactive iodine should usually be the last resort:

Reason #1: Receiving radioactive iodine will most likely make you hypothyroid for the rest of your life. Because radioactive iodine obliterates the thyroid gland, most people will develop hypothyroidism. As a result, most of these people will need to take thyroid hormone for the rest of their life. While many people do fine on thyroid hormone, why damage or destroy your thyroid gland if you don't have to? The thyroid gland is one of the most important parts of the body, and shouldn't be obliterated or removed unless absolutely necessary.

Reason #2: Many people do fine while taking antithyroid drugs. When I spoke with an endocrinologist upon being diagnosed with Graves' Disease, she was somewhat conservative, and she didn't recommend radioactive iodine to me. Instead she prescribed antithyroid drugs, which I didn't take, but I did respect her for not being too aggressive right off the bat. Even though antithyroid drugs won't cure hyperthyroidism or Graves' Disease, in my opinion it's definitely a better first option when compared to radioactive iodine. Plus, antithyroid drugs do a good job of managing the symptoms in many people. Some people actually will go into a state of remission while taking antithyroid drugs, although this usually is temporary. But many people who won't even consider natural treatment methods have done well for years taking antithyroid drugs.

In fact, studies show that hyperthyroidism can be controlled with antithyroid drugs with only rare exceptions. Could this be the reason why many endocrinologists who practice outside of the United States recommend antithyroid medication first, and perhaps explain why some endocrinologists in the United States are strongly opposed to radioactive iodine treatment? Of course some people don't respond well when taking antithyroid medication, and some people have allergies to this medication and therefore are unable to take it. While I realize that not everyone can have their symptoms managed through antithyroid medication, to not at least attempt to manage the person's symptoms in this manner before recommending a treatment that damages their thyroid gland is ludicrous.

Reason #3: Radioactive iodine doesn't do anything for the underlying cause of the disorder. While radioactive iodine will usually eliminate the hyperthyroid symptoms, this harsh treatment method doesn't do anything for the actual cause of the disorder. This of course is why I recommend natural treatment methods, as my goal is to always try to get to the underlying cause of the person's condition. And since the malfunctioning thyroid gland isn't the actual cause of the problem in most cases, many people who receive radioactive iodine will develop other health issues in the future.

If becoming permanently hypothyroid isn't enough to discourage you from receiving radioactive iodine, then how about this piece of research: "long-term follow-up studies have revealed an increased cardiovascular mortality in those with a past history of hyperthyroidism treated with RAI".[27]

Another study showed that "Among patients with hyperthyroidism treated with radioiodine, mortality from all causes and mortality due to cardiovascular and cerebrovascular disease and fracture are increased".[28]

Why Can't Endocrinologists Agree Which Treatment Method Is The Best?

What's amazing is that endocrinologists can't even agree with regards to which treatment methods patients should receive. When I was doing my research for this book, I came across various different opinions, and here is an example of the opinions held by four different endocrinologists:[29]

"I treat almost everyone with propylthiouracil. I avoid 131I in all patients unless there are reasons to the contrary. I have not recommended surgery in 15 years for such patients."

"All my patients are given the option of selecting 131I, surgery, or antithyroid drugs. I advise 131I as the simplest, safest, cheapest, decisive treatment. Ninety percent accept this advice".

"There is no question that time and experience world-wide have shown that 131I is the treatment of choice for thyrotoxicosis"

"We remain conservative with regard to radioiodine in patients of childbearing and child-siring age. Because of the persistence of leukocyte chromosomal breakage for years after radioidine therapy, we would like to see the F1 generation assurances of the safety of radioiodine".

When Is Radioactive Iodine Really Necessary?

So when is radioactive iodine treatment really necessary to receive? Here are two of the primary situations when radioactive iodine might truly be necessary:

1. **When Every Other Treatment Option Has Failed.** In most cases, people with hyperthyroidism and Graves' Disease should choose to take antithyroid drugs to manage the symptoms before receiving radioactive iodine. Although these prescription drugs won't cure hyperthyroidism or Graves' Disease, they usually do a good job of managing the symptoms, might lower the thyroid antibodies, and sometimes will put a person into a state of remission, although most of the time it's temporary. But in most cases this option is definitely better than obliterating your thyroid gland.

   I of course recommend natural treatment methods to people, as while not everyone can be helped through natural treatment methods, many people can have their health restored back to normal. It admittedly is a challenge to follow such a protocol, which is a reason why some people choose antithyroid drugs, and even radioactive iodine. After all, it's much easier to take medication daily or receive the radioactive iodine treatment than to follow a natural treatment protocol. But when you think about how important the thyroid gland is to your health, it is well worth making the "sacrifice" to restore your health back to normal.

If you have taken antithyroid drugs and followed a natural treatment protocol, and if you still have moderate to severe hyperthyroid symptoms, then in this situation it might be necessary to receive radioactive iodine. Of course this would mean you're not responding to the antithyroid drugs, and you completely followed the recommendations of the natural endocrine doctor, yet the natural treatment methods didn't do the job either. One problem is that we live in an impatient society, and many people who follow a natural treatment protocol expect quick results. And while one frequently notices changes in the symptoms after a few weeks, it will usually take months to completely eliminate a person's symptoms. And it will take even longer until the blood tests normalize.

2. **Certain Cases Of Thyroid Cancer.** Some people with thyroid cancer will need to receive radioactive iodine. But how does someone with thyroid cancer know if it is really necessary to receive RAI? Well, this is a situation that most holistic doctors probably would stay away from. So what I would recommend is to seek the opinion of a second, or even a third endocrinologist to be certain of this.

Just remember that even if radioactive iodine treatment is necessary, this still doesn't correct the cause of the problem. Whether someone developed primary hyperthyroidism, or thyroid cancer, there still were factors which led to the development of these conditions. This is why it's not a bad idea for someone who received RAI to consult with a holistic doctor. Frequently such people are just told to take thyroid hormone for the rest of their life after receiving radioactive iodine (for those that become hypothyroid). Thyroid hormone sometimes does a great job of managing the symptoms, but many people still have moderate to severe symptoms, even when taking synthetic or natural thyroid hormone for their hypothyroid condition. Just remember that RAI doesn't do anything for the immune system component of Graves' Disease, doesn't address compromised adrenal glands which may be an issue, and definitely won't correct any existing imbalances of the sex hormones, which also can play a role in hyperthyroid conditions.

So there are definitely situations when someone needs to receive radioactive iodine. I realize it can be tough to make a decision when an endocrinologist tells you that RAI is necessary. But one shouldn't take obliteration of their thyroid gland lightly. As a result, if a doctor recommends that you receive radioactive iodine and you're not sure if this is the right decision, consider what I have discussed, and if necessary, receive a second opinion. After all, you only have one thyroid gland, and you want to do everything you can to keep it if at all possible.

Still Skeptical About the Risks Of Radioactive Iodine? Then Please Read The Following:

For those who still are skeptical about the risks of radioactive iodine, keep in mind that those who receive radioactive iodine are instructed to take certain precautions the first few days after receiving this treatment. This includes using separate towels and bed linens, different plates and silverware, etc. They are also advised to sleep in a separate bed from their partner, and to avoid kissing and sexual intercourse for a few days after receiving radioactive iodine. Some will advise people who have received radioactive iodine treatment to flush the toilet a few times after using the bathroom in order to dilute the amount of radiation in the urine and feces. In some countries, people who receive radioactive iodine are actually quarantined for a few days. Remember that this is radiation we're talking about, and so while some people might need to receive this treatment method, any medical doctor who claims that it's completely harmless is either naive or is being dishonest.

Can Someone Benefit From Natural Treatment Methods AFTER Receiving Radioactive Iodine?

Some people who have already received radioactive iodine wonder whether they would benefit from natural treatment methods. Unfortunately this isn't an easy question to answer, as it really does depend on the extent of damage which was done to the thyroid gland. The good news is that just because you received radioactive iodine treatment doesn't mean you can't benefit from natural treatment methods. This is true even if you have become hypothyroid as a result of this harsh treatment procedure.

The reason for this is because the body has an amazing ability to heal. While a person who has a thyroid gland that was completely removed through surgery or one that was damaged extensively through RAI very well might need to take thyroid hormone for the rest of their life, partial damage or partial removal of this gland still offers some hope of being able to restore your health through a natural treatment protocol.

Many people who have received radioactive iodine become depressed and sometimes even angry when they realize that they might have had a chance to "save" their thyroid gland instead of permanently damaging it through this treatment. But once again, if you received radioactive iodine treatment you still might be able to be helped through natural treatment methods. In fact, the question really isn't whether or not you can benefit from natural treatment methods, but whether or not you can have your thyroid health restored back to normal. As for completely restoring your thyroid health, this admittedly is more difficult to accomplish after receiving radioactive iodine, although sometimes it still is possible depending on the amount of damage which was done to the thyroid gland.

For those people who received radioactive iodine and can't have their health restored through a natural treatment protocol, they still can usually benefit from natural treatment methods. The reason for this is because radioactive iodine does nothing for the actual cause of the hyperthyroid condition. While it does usually help manage the symptoms, just remember that in most cases the malfunctioning thyroid gland isn't the cause of the hyperthyroid disorder, as I have mentioned numerous times already.

So as you know by now, the goal of a natural treatment protocol is not just to manage your symptoms, but to get to the underlying cause of the disorder. Sometimes natural treatment methods will be able to restore the health of the individual who has received radioactive iodine. Other times it's not possible to completely restore their thyroid health, but it is still is important to restore the health of other areas of their body which led to the development of their disorder, which will help to prevent future conditions from developing.

As for how someone who received radioactive iodine can know for certain whether or not they can have their health restored back to normal through natural treatment methods, unfortunately there really is no surefire way to know this. The only way to truly determine whether someone who has received radioactive iodine can be helped through natural treatment methods is to actually give these treatment methods a try. The good news is that it usually doesn't take too long to see if these treatment methods are helping.

Getting Over The Anger Of Receiving Radioactive Iodine

As I briefly mentioned previously, after learning that a natural treatment protocol can potentially help with a hyperthyroid condition, some people become upset, and even angry that they received radioactive iodine treatment. If this describes you, I can understand your frustration. The truth is that while radioactive iodine should be used as a last resort, what you need to understand is that this is how most endocrinologists and other medical doctors are trained to treat such conditions.

While there are some great endocrinologists in practice, most are trained to use drugs and radioactive iodine treatment as their primary treatment methods for hyperthyroid conditions. In fact, if you were to ask your endocrinologist or general medical practitioner about natural treatment methods, chances are they would advise you not to follow through with such a protocol.

As I have already mentioned in this book, even though I'm a holistic doctor, I honestly was skeptical before I received natural treatment methods for Graves' Disease. And who knows whether my condition is completely cured, or in a state of remission. All I know is that I'm feeling great and have no regrets about the choices I have made. But for those people who have already received radioactive iodine treatment, please don't give up hope. There still is a chance that the function of your thyroid gland can be restored through a natural treatment protocol. It admittedly will be more challenging when compared with someone who hasn't received radioactive iodine, but restoring your health is still a possibility. And even if this isn't the case, just remember that what originally caused your hyperthyroid condition to develop probably still exists. Because of this, at the very least you should consider natural treatment methods to "optimize" your health and to prevent other conditions from developing in the future.

Chapter Summary

- The following represent three reasons why radioactive iodine should usually be the last resort: 1) Receiving radioactive iodine will most likely make you hypothyroid for the rest of your life. 2) Some people do fine while taking antithyroid drugs , and 3) radioactive iodine doesn't do anything for the underlying cause of the disorder.
- Here are two of the primary situations when radioactive iodine treatment might truly be necessary: 1) When every other treatment option has failed and 2) with certain cases of thyroid cancer
- Just because you received radioactive iodine therapy doesn't mean you can't benefit from natural treatment methods.
- The only way to truly determine whether someone who has received radioactive iodine therapy can be helped through natural treatment methods is to actually give them a try. The good news is that it usually doesn't take too long to see if these treatment methods are helping.

For more information on these and other natural thyroid health topics, visit www.GravesDiseaseBook.com

CHAPTER 17

The Risks Of Playing The Waiting Game

WHEN BELINDA WAS diagnosed with Graves' Disease by her endocrinologist, the doctor was conservative and didn't recommend radioactive iodine. Instead, she told Belinda to take Methimazole to manage the hyperthyroid symptoms. Her advice was to take the Methimazole for 18 months, and to see if it goes into a state of remission. Belinda took the Methimazole, and sure enough, her Graves' Disease condition went into remission, and after the 18 months had passed she was able to stop taking the antithyroid medication.

Of course the antithyroid drugs didn't do anything for the underlying cause of the disorder, so it shouldn't have been a surprise when about eight months later she began experiencing hyperthyroid symptoms again. Belinda went back to her endocrinologist, who surprisingly put her back on the Methimazole, but warned Belinda that she might need to receive radioactive iodine to permanently "fix" the problem. At the time Belinda was an email subscriber on my website, and after reading some of my articles and watching some of the videos on my website she decided it would be a good idea to schedule a consultation with me. To make a long story short, upon following a natural treatment protocol Belinda's symptoms subsided in about one month, her thyroid blood levels normalized after four months, and she learned how to maintain her health in order to prevent a relapse from occurring.

Many people with hyperthyroidism and Graves' Disease who don't receive radioactive iodine will take antithyroid medication. Taking antithyroid drugs definitely is a more conservative option than receiving radioactive iodine. And for many people, antithyroid drugs do a good job of managing their hyperthyroid symptoms. PTU and Methimazole are two of the more popular antithyroid drugs taken by many people with hyperthyroidism and Graves' Disease.

Taking antithyroid medication can be wise with someone who has hyperthyroidism or Graves' Disease. After all, hyperthyroid symptoms can at times be severe, and it's risky to deal with a very high pulse rate, severe palpitations, etc. So without question, some people do need to take antithyroid drugs to help manage their symptoms.

Antithyroid Drugs Are Usually A Temporary Solution

While antithyroid drugs will usually help to manage someone's hyperthyroid symptoms, in my opinion they should only be used on a temporary basis in the majority of cases. Of course for someone who is not looking to follow a natural treatment protocol, then perhaps this is the best long term option. The problem is that many people take antithyroid drugs and pray their condition will go into a state of remission. While some people do go into a state of remission when taking antithyroid drugs, many people don't. Plus, many people who do go into a state of remission will eventually relapse in the future. So what may happen is that someone who is taking antithyroid drugs for one or two years may go into a state of remission, but after a few months or years the hyperthyroid symptoms can return, and when this happens they will most likely end up receiving radioactive iodine to obliterate their thyroid gland.

Of course the reason for the relapse is because the cause of the condition was never addressed. Once again, the antithyroid drugs may do a good job of managing the symptoms, but they won't do anything to cure the actual condition. So the person who takes these drugs and goes into a state of remission but then never addresses the actual cause will never be cured of their condition.

It's Risky To Aim For A Remission Through Taking Drugs

In a different chapter I spoke about the difference between remission and cure, and I discussed how someone with hyperthyroidism or Graves' Disease might suffer a relapse, even if they restore their health back to normal through natural treatment methods. Because of this, you might wonder what's the difference between suffering a relapse when taking antithyroid drugs when compared to following a natural treatment protocol? After all, it's easy to take medication, but can be very challenging to follow a natural treatment protocol. Plus, if someone follows a natural treatment protocol, neglects their health, and suffers a relapse, they probably will need to follow another natural treatment protocol.

However, one has to consider a few things. First of all, antithyroid drugs don't always effectively manage the symptoms. And even if they do manage the hyperthyroid symptoms, many people feel lousy when taking antithyroid drugs. The second thing a person needs to consider is that antithyroid drugs don't do anything for the actual cause of the disorder.

So for example, even if someone with a hyperthyroid condition who has weak adrenal glands and a compromised immune system responds well while taking antithyroid drugs, this isn't doing anything for compromised adrenal glands and immune system.

So not only is someone who goes into remission very likely to relapse, but this person has a good chance of developing other autoimmune conditions, as I explained in a previous chapter. So in this example it would be important for them to address both the adrenal glands and the immune system component. Similarly, if they had digestive issues or any hormone imbalances, taking antithyroid drugs wouldn't do anything to help with these conditions.

If You're Looking For A Quick Cure...

Without question it is more challenging to follow a natural treatment protocol than to take prescription drugs. When I conduct my free webinars on natural thyroid health (you can find out more about these free webinars on my website), I always mention how people who aren't willing to take responsibility for their health shouldn't bother speaking with a natural endocrine doctor. I wish it were an easy process, but the truth is that it takes many years for conditions such as hyperthyroidism and Graves' Disease to develop, so it's ridiculous to expect a quick and easy cure.

Antithyroid drugs can provide a quicker solution to manage the symptoms when following a natural treatment protocol. But by no means should they be looked at as being a cure. Some people are happy with taking antithyroid drugs, which is fine. However, if you're looking to address the actual cause of your disorder and would like to attempt to restore your health back to normal, which I'm guessing you're interested in since you're reading this book, then you should strongly consider following a natural treatment protocol.

Chapter Summary

- While antithyroid drugs can help manage someone's hyperthyroid symptoms, in my opinion they should only be used on a temporary basis in most cases.

- While some people do go into a state of remission when taking antithyroid drugs, many people don't. Plus, many people who do go into a state of remission will eventually relapse in the future.

- Not only is someone who goes into remission very likely to relapse, but there is a risk of other autoimmune conditions developing in the future

- The truth is that it takes many years for conditions such as hyperthyroidism and Graves' Disease to develop, so it's ridiculous to expect a quick cure.

For more information on these and other natural thyroid health topics, visit www.GravesDiseaseBook.com

CHAPTER 18

Combining Natural Treatment Methods With Conventional Treatment Methods

TERRI WAS INTERESTED in following a natural treatment protocol, but she was concerned about stopping her thyroid medication. By reading some of the articles I have written she realized that I have no problem with someone following a natural treatment protocol while taking the antithyroid drugs. When I consulted with her for the first time I told her that it would be fine for her to take the antithyroid medication while beginning the natural treatment protocol, and that only she can make the decision to wean off the antithyroid drugs.

And that's exactly what happened, as she felt better upon following the natural treatment protocol, and she advised her endocrinologist that she was going to reduce the dosage until she had completely weaned off of the antithyroid medication. The endocrinologist wasn't happy to hear this, and told her that the natural treatment protocol wouldn't correct the problem, and she would eventually need to take the antithyroid medication again or receive radioactive iodine. Well, Terri successfully weaned herself off of the drugs, and because she continues to maintain her health she continues to feel great to this day.

Some people are hesitant to give natural treatment methods a try because they are concerned about stopping the prescription medication they are taking for their hyperthyroid condition. Being a holistic doctor I will never tell any patient to stop taking antithyroid drugs. I might tell someone my story about when I was diagnosed with Graves' Disease and how I personally decided not to take any antithyroid medication. But I will never tell anyone to stop taking their medication, as this is only a decision they can make on their own. In fact, there are times when I think it's a good idea for people with hyperthyroid conditions to take the antithyroid drugs on a temporary basis to help manage their symptoms. But ultimately it's up to the patient to decide what they want to do.

So for those people who want to give natural treatment methods a try but at the same time want to continue taking their current medication, there is no rule which says they can't continue taking antithyroid drugs and still follow a natural treatment protocol. Of course there might be some contraindications regarding certain supplements and herbs which normally would be recommended if you weren't taking any prescription drugs, but any good holistic doctor should be able to advise the patient what they can and cannot take while taking thyroid medication.

When I was diagnosed with Graves' Disease, I had the option of taking the antithyroid drugs and the beta blocker, and then I still could have began the natural treatment protocol. If I took this approach then once the symptoms were under control and I was following the natural treatment protocol for a few months I could have weaned myself off of the drugs, and then let the natural treatment protocol take over. This definitely was an option I considered, but I decided to not take the antithyroid drugs or beta blocker and I just followed a natural treatment protocol, which turned out to be a great decision on my part.

What Is The Best Option For You?

As far as what you should do, once again, this is a decision that only you can make. I will say that I think people with a hyperthyroid condition are more at risk when they don't manage their symptoms when compared with someone who has hypothyroidism, and therefore they might want to consider taking antithyroid drugs if their symptoms are severe. So for someone who has a very high pulse rate and severe palpitations, it might be a good idea to take the antithyroid drugs and/or a beta blocker, and then follow the natural treatment protocol while weaning themselves off of the drugs. This again is just an option, as I'm not trying to recommend that anyone who has been diagnosed with a hyperthyroid condition should make this choice.

As I briefly mentioned earlier, for some people with a hyperthyroid condition, it's actually a good idea for them to continue taking their antithyroid medication while beginning the natural treatment protocol. Even though fatalities with hyperthyroidism and Graves' Disease are rare, it does happen from time to time, and anyone who has a high pulse rate or any other cardiac symptoms really should try to manage them. If you're currently not taking antithyroid drugs then the question that probably comes to your mind is "how high should my pulse rate be before I decide to take antithyroid drugs?" There is no specific answer to this, as all I can say is that people with moderate to severe symptoms definitely need to manage their symptoms.

Are Bugleweed & Motherwort Good Substitutes For Antithyroid Drugs?

In the chapter where I spoke about nutritional supplements and herbs, I spoke about the herbs Bugleweed and Motherwort, and how they can help a great deal with the symptoms in many people with hyperthyroidism and Graves' Disease. And there are many people who decide not to take the antithyroid drugs, but instead take one or both of these herbs. However, while these herbs are great, sometimes they aren't enough to control a person's hyperthyroid symptoms, especially if they are severe. This is especially true with emergency situations such as thyroid storm, as someone with this condition definitely shouldn't rely on herbs to manage their symptoms.

But even when the symptoms aren't considered to be life threatening, which is the case with most people who have a hyperthyroid condition, you do need to be careful about just taking these or any other herbs as substitutes for antithyroid drugs. I'm of course not suggesting that these herbs aren't effective, as I used them to manage my hyperthyroid symptoms when I was diagnosed with Graves' Disease, and many of my patients use them to manage their hyperthyroid symptoms as well. All I'm trying to say is that they shouldn't be viewed as a substitute for antithyroid drugs, as for some people looking to follow a natural treatment protocol, the antithyroid drugs might do a better job of managing the person's symptoms until the natural treatment protocol begins to take effect. This is just something you need to keep in mind, as while both Bugleweed and Motherwort work well for many people with hyperthyroidism and Graves' Disease, I've also had patients who took both Bugleweed and Motherwort and who didn't notice much of difference in their symptoms after taking these herbs for some time. This doesn't mean the herbs aren't effective, but for some people they aren't potent enough to effectively manage the symptoms.

Taking Antithyroid Medication For A Prolonged Period Of Time

Some people actually choose to take the antithyroid medication for the amount of time their medical doctor recommended and at the same time follow the natural treatment protocol. In other words, they don't wean off of the antithyroid drugs a few months into the natural treatment protocol, but they instead take the medication for as long as they were told to by their doctor. For example, if they were told to take PTU or Methimazole for 18 months, then some will take it for the full 18 months, and at the same time follow a natural treatment protocol. While most of the people I consult with don't want to take the antithyroid drugs for a prolonged period of time, I have no problem consulting with someone who chooses this option.

It's Best To Consult With Your Endocrinologist or General Medical Practitioner

Whenever someone with hyperthyroidism or Graves' Disease consults with me and is taking antithyroid medication, I always give them the different options they have, and then tell them they should discuss these options with their endocrinologist or medical doctor. In my opinion, no holistic doctor should tell any patient to stop taking any prescription drugs they are currently taking, unless perhaps if they happen to be a holistic medical doctor. So to play it safe I always refer the patient back to their primary care physician just so it is known that it wasn't I who made the decision for the patient to stop taking their medication, but instead it was a decision made between the patient and their medical doctor.

With that being said, many medical doctors, including most endocrinologists, won't approve of any patient following a natural treatment protocol. As a result, I let the patient know that while they should consult with their medical doctor about the different options they have, there is a good chance their doctor won't approve of them following such a protocol. And a big reason for this is because they don't have a good knowledge about natural treatment methods, and most don't want to open their minds to these methods. This of course doesn't describe every medical doctor, as fortunately there are some holistic medical doctors who understand how safe and effective natural treatment methods can be.

In any case, it is the person with the hyperthyroid condition who needs to make this decision as to whether they should stop taking the prescription medication, or continue taking drugs while following a natural treatment protocol. Even if they speak with an endocrinologist or another type of medical doctor who is open to natural treatment methods, it ultimately is the patient who will need to make the decision. The goal of the holistic healthcare professional is to give the patient all of the information they need in order to make an informed decision, and not to make the actual decision for the patient.

To summarize this chapter, for anyone with hyperthyroidism or Graves' Disease who is currently taking antithyroid drugs, or is considering taking them, it is fine to combine both conventional and natural treatment methods. Taking the prescription drugs won't prevent you from restoring your health back to normal, and in fact could be important if your hyperthyroid symptoms are severe. While many people want to try to avoid taking any type of medication if at all possible, at the same time you need to be smart about this, as you really need to weigh the benefits and risks in this situation.

Chapter Summary

- For those people who want to give natural treatment methods a try but at the same time want to continue taking their current medication, there is no rule which says they can't continue taking antithyroid drugs and still follow a natural treatment protocol.

- For someone who has a high pulse rate and severe palpitations, it might be a good idea to take the antithyroid drugs and/or a beta blocker, and then follow the natural treatment protocol while weaning themselves off of the drugs under the supervision of their endocrinologist.

- Although the herbs Bugleweed and Motherwort can do an excellent job of managing a person's symptoms, they shouldn't be viewed as a substitute for antithyroid drugs for people with severe hyperthyroid symptoms.

- It is the person with the hyperthyroid condition who needs to make this decision as to whether they should stop taking drugs, or continue taking drugs while following a natural treatment protocol.

For more information on these and other natural thyroid health topics, visit www.GravesDiseaseBook.com

CHAPTER 19

Can Natural Treatment Methods Help With Thyroid Nodules?

SOME PEOPLE WITH hyperthyroidism and Graves' Disease have thyroid nodules, which are abnormal growths of thyroid tissue. In most cases, thyroid nodules aren't anything to be concerned about, but sometimes they can cause problems which need to be addressed. Many times endocrinologists will recommend that a person with thyroid nodules take extreme actions, even when they aren't causing any issues. So the goal of this chapter is to discuss some of the situations where it may be necessary to intervene, and other situations when it is best to leave the thyroid nodules alone.

The following are situations when someone with a hyperthyroid condition who has thyroid nodules should consider using medical intervention:

1. **If the thyroid nodule is malignant.** If the thyroid nodule is malignant, then this is an obvious situation which requires medical intervention. Less than 1% of all thyroid nodules are malignant,[30] which is of course good news. If the nodule is cold on the radioactive iodine uptake scan then there is a greater chance of it being malignant. But the majority of these are also benign as well.[31] In order to determine if a nodule is cancerous, a fine needle aspiration is required. If the thyroid nodule is found to be malignant, then surgery of the thyroid nodule and/or the thyroid gland itself will most likely be recommended.

2. **When there is a physical obstruction caused by the thyroid nodule.** If the thyroid nodule is causing an obstruction, leading to difficulty with swallowing and/or breathing, then this is another obvious example of where medical intervention is required. Once again, in these situations, surgical removal of the thyroid nodule or the actual thyroid gland is usually recommended

3. **If the thyroid nodule is causing excess secretion of thyroid hormone.** If hyperthyroidism results due to one or more thyroid nodules, then this is yet another reason why medical intervention might be required. While radioactive iodine therapy or surgery is frequently recommended under these circumstances, another option is to take antithyroid drugs to control the symptoms, and then at the same time follow a natural thyroid treatment protocol in an attempt to shrink the thyroid nodule. Even though this approach isn't always effective, in my opinion it's definitely worth giving it a try in order to possibly prevent thyroid surgery.

4. **When there is any other pain or discomfort due to the presence of the thyroid nodule.** If the thyroid nodule is causing any type of pain or physical discomfort, then medical intervention will most likely be required. This is yet another scenario where surgical removal of the thyroid nodule is usually recommended.

Is Surgery Of The Thyroid Gland Really Necessary?

For many of these problems involving thyroid nodules, surgery of the thyroid gland itself will be recommended. While surgery will most likely resolve the problems previously listed, there are potential risks involved with thyroid surgery. One risk is that the person is most likely to become hypothyroid, especially if the entire thyroid gland is removed. But even with a partial thyroidectomy there still is a chance the person can become hypothyroid. If this happens then they will be advised to take synthetic or natural thyroid hormone for the rest of their life.

Of course in some cases, complete removal of the thyroid gland might be necessary. But if at all possible, removal of the thyroid nodule alone would be a much better option. This not only will take care of the problem, but will also leave much of the thyroid gland intact, which is the ideal scenario. Even though there still is the chance of the person becoming hypothyroid in this situation, there is also the chance they won't develop hypothyroidism, and therefore won't need to take thyroid hormone for the rest of their life.

Another potential risk of receiving surgery of the thyroid gland is that it can cause damage to some of the surrounding structures, including the parathyroid glands and the larynx. These problems are more common than you would think, and is yet another reason why thyroid gland surgery should be avoided if at all possible. Once again, I realize this isn't always possible, but if your endocrinologist tells you that surgery of the thyroid gland is necessary, you probably will want to receive a second opinion.

Of course I am not an endocrinologist, nor am I a surgeon, and so I can't tell you why many times they opt to remove the entire thyroid gland, rather than just remove the thyroid nodule itself. Actually, one of the main reasons is because many people who receive a partial thyroidec-tomy will become hypothyroid, as I just mentioned before. But as I also just mentioned, not everyone who receives a partial thyroidectomy will develop hypothyroidism.

Just as is the case with radioactive iodine, many endocrinologists can't agree with one another with regards to the approach to take with thyroid nodules. To no surprise, studies show that surgeons are more in favor of surgery of thyroid nodules when compared to non-surgeons. Another study showed that "only malignant or large symptomatic nodules require surgical excision". The same study showed that "fine-needle aspiration, biopsy, guided by ultrasonography when possible, results in substantial reduction of unnecessary surgery".[32] In other words, some surgeries can be prevented simply by doing thorough testing.

Can Natural Thyroid Treatment Methods Help Prevent Surgery?

Is it possible to use natural thyroid treatment methods to shrink the thyroid nodule, and thus avoid surgery? Well, the problem is that some of these cases require immediate intervention. And if natural treat-ment methods were successful in shrinking the thyroid nodule, this still takes time to accomplish. Someone with a serious obstruction probably wouldn't be able to wait for the effects of the natural treatment methods to take place. So while following a natural thyroid treatment protocol might help to shrink the thyroid nodule over time, in some cases imme-diate intervention is necessary.

On the other hand, if you have problems due to a thyroid nodule which aren't too severe, then it very well might be worth giving natural treat-ment methods a try. For example, many endocrinologists recommend surgery, even when the patient's symptoms aren't too severe. But assuming the symptoms aren't severe, then you really don't have much to lose by following a natural treatment protocol. And taking this approach can potentially help preserve your thyroid gland and allow you to avoid taking thyroid hormone for the rest of your life. So I do recommend natural thyroid treatment methods in cases where the thyroid nodule isn't malignant, and isn't causing an obstruction or any severe symptoms.

Of course some people want a guarantee that their thyroid nodule can be shrunk by following a natural treatment protocol. Obviously no doctor can make such a guarantee, as it's not as if there is some "magic" supplement or herb which will shrink thyroid nodules. But by following a natural thyroid treatment protocol and balancing the person's thyroid hormone levels, sometimes this problem will self-resolve. And let's not forget that following a natural treatment protocol won't just help benefit your thyroid health, but your overall health as well. So even if you follow a natural treatment protocol but it doesn't shrink any thyroid nodules you may have, it's not as if following the protocol was a complete waste, as it will benefit your health in many other ways.

In summary, if you have hyperthyroidism or Graves' Disease, along with one or more thyroid nodules, and have been told by your endocrinologist that surgery to remove the nodule or thyroid gland itself is necessary, it's a good idea to obtain a second opinion. And if you aren't experiencing severe symptoms, then you very well might want to consider speaking with a competent natural endocrine doctor to see if natural treatment methods might be able to help you. While there are no guarantees that such a protocol can shrink your thyroid nodule, it is a much more conservative approach than receiving surgery, radioactive iodine, or any other extreme medical procedures. And of course if the natural treatment protocol is successful in shrinking the thyroid nodule it will most likely help you to avoid thyroid surgery or RAI.

Chapter Summary

- Many times endocrinologists will recommend that a person with thyroid nodules take extreme actions, even when they aren't causing any issues.
- The following are situations when someone with a hyperthyroid condition who has thyroid nodules should consider choosing medical intervention: 1) if the thyroid nodule is malignant, 2) when there is a physical obstruction caused by the thyroid nodule, 3) if the thyroid nodule is causing excess secretion of thyroid hormone, 4) when there is any other pain or discomfort due to the presence of the thyroid nodule
- In some cases, partial or complete removal of the thyroid gland might be necessary. But if at all possible, removal of the thyroid nodule alone would be a much better option.
- Even if you follow a natural treatment protocol but it doesn't shrink any thyroid nodules you have, it's not as if following the protocol was a complete waste, as it will benefit your health in many other ways.

For more information on these and other natural thyroid health topics, visit www.GravesDiseaseBook.com

CHAPTER 20

Overcoming Thyroid Eye Disease

THYROID EYE DISEASE, also known as Graves' ophthalmopathy, is an inflammatory eye condition which affects a small percentage of people with Graves' Disease, as well as some people with Hashimoto's Thyroiditis. It involves the same antibodies which attack the thyroid gland, as these antibodies can also attack the tissues of the eyes. Of those people this condition does affect, only a small percentage will have severe symptoms. The good news is that this condition will self-resolve in most people, but it still can cause long-lasting problems, most commonly exophthalmos (bulging eyes).

Although this condition usually self-resolves, sometimes conventional medical treatment is necessary to help manage the symptoms. For example, corticosteroids are used in some cases to help with the inflammation. And in some cases more extreme treatment methods are used, such as radiation, immunosuppressant drugs, and sometimes even surgery.

Natural Thyroid Treatment Methods To The Rescue?

Can natural thyroid treatment methods cure thyroid eye disease, or prevent it from developing in someone who currently isn't stricken with this condition? Let's first answer the second question. If someone has Graves' Disease and is following a natural treatment protocol, and if this is successful in restoring their health back to normal then in most cases the person won't develop thyroid eye disease. And even if following such a protocol doesn't completely restore their health back to normal, since this protocol will help to address the immune system and optimize their overall health, there still is a good chance it will prevent the occurrence of thyroid eye disease. This once again is based on the experience I have had with my patients.

On the other hand, for someone who already has thyroid eye disease, natural treatment methods still can usually help. This doesn't mean that natural treatment methods will always help with thyroid eye disease, and it is definitely more challenging with severe cases. For example, if someone has a severe case of exophthalmos, following a natural treatment protocol may not completely reverse this. Does this mean that someone with severe symptoms shouldn't follow a natural treatment protocol? Not necessarily, as while there are cases where such a protocol can't fully restore the health of someone with thyroid eye disease, in many cases it can help greatly, or at the very least manage the symptoms without the person having to worry about the side effects which are common with conventional medical treatment. So while there are no guarantees, it definitely is worth a try in my opinion.

The Risks Of Receiving Radioactive Iodine Treatment With Thyroid Eye Disease

Some studies show that radioactive iodine therapy is associated with an increased risk of thyroid eye disease,[33] although this doesn't happen in all patients who receive RAI. Anyone who has visited my website knows that I'm not a big fan of radioactive iodine (and you of course realize this by reading this book). This is true even when people don't have thyroid eye disease. While some people do need to receive radioactive iodine, it usually should be a last resort, after everything else has been tried. So whether or not you have thyroid eye disease, in my biased opinion I would highly recommend that you at least consider giving natural thyroid treatment methods a try first, unless if it's a medical emergency which requires you receiving radioactive iodine.

For those people who do receive radioactive iodine treatment and experience an increase in their thyroid eye disease symptoms, in most cases corticosteroids will be recommended. If you have thyroid eye disease and have received RAI, and are now experiencing a worsening of your symptoms, you might wonder at this point whether or not natural treatment methods would be effective. Even with people who have received radioactive iodine treatment, natural thyroid treatment methods can potentially help. While it is less likely that someone who has received radioactive iodine therapy can have their health restored back to normal, some people can have their health restored if their thyroid gland wasn't completely obliterated, and many others who can't have their health restored still can benefit greatly from following such a protocol.

A Summary Of The Different Treatment Options You Have With Thyroid Eye Disease

Treatment Option #1: Conventional Medical Treatment. As mentioned before, there are numerous medical treatment approaches depending on your condition. Many people with this condition are prescribed steroids to help with the inflammation. Others with severe symptoms might receive more aggressive treatment procedures. I'm not going to sit here and criticize these medical treatments, as sometimes they can do a good job of managing the symptoms, which no doubt is important. On the other hand, just like any other type of medical treatment, they can also lead to numerous side effects. So if you do choose the medical treatment option, just keep in mind that this usually is just a temporary solution, although this might be fine since many times this condition will self resolve anyway.

Treatment Option #2: Natural Treatment Methods. I'm obviously biased towards using a holistic treatment approach, as my goal is always to try to get to the root cause of the problem. Once again, I do think symptom management is important, and because of this, sometimes it is necessary to take prescription drugs. However, in my opinion this should be temporary if at all possible, as if one chooses a natural treatment protocol and at the same time takes medication to control their symptoms, then I see nothing wrong with this. On the other hand, for those people who simply take the advice of their medical doctor without wanting to try to restore their health back to normal, I'd be lying if I told you that this doesn't frustrate me.

I realize that many people are skeptical when it comes to both the safety and effectiveness of natural treatment methods. I just wonder why they aren't just as worried about the potential short-term and long-term side effects of the conventional medical treatment methods. When following a natural treatment protocol, in most cases the worst case scenario involves the person not responding. With regards to receiving medical treatment, the worst case scenario is usually an extreme exacerbation of their symptoms. Actually, it can be worse than this, as there is always the risk of fatalities when receiving any type of surgery, and even when taking corticosteroids, although in the latter case it usually takes years for these drugs to lead to serious health issues which can cause death. But my point is that there is usually very little risk in treating your thyroid eye disease condition naturally under the guidance of a competent holistic doctor, but there can be substantial risks with taking the medical route.

Treatment Option #3: Combining Conventional & Natural Treatment Methods. As I briefly mentioned earlier, and also spoke about in detail in a previous chapter, this is an option I have nothing against. Some people want to try to restore their health back to normal, but at the same time want to take medication to help manage their symptoms until the natural treatment methods "kick in". As I mentioned earlier, when dealing with a condition such as Graves' Disease, not only am I supportive of this approach, but in many cases I would actually recommend it. My concern is not so much the progression of the thyroid eye disease, but rather that the symptoms of hyperthyroidism and Graves' Disease itself can become dangerous, specifically the increased heart rate and heart palpitations.

Treatment Option #4: No Treatment. Since many cases of thyroid eye disease will self resolve without any intervention, this is yet another option you have. Many people will choose to receive no treatment, especially if their symptoms are mild. If this is the case, you might decide not to choose either medical or natural treatment methods, and hope that the condition goes away on its own and doesn't become any worse.

In summary, thyroid eye disease is a condition that is rare, and when it does affect someone, the symptoms are usually mild and warrant minimal or no treatment. However, in cases where the symptoms are moderate or severe, medical treatment might be able to help manage the symptoms, but you might want to consider a natural treatment protocol to get to the underlying cause of this condition. This of course not only will help with the symptoms, but even if your health can be completely restored to normal, natural treatment methods still can prevent the condition from progressing in many people. If you want more information on this condition, the best book I have read so far on this topic is called "Thyroid Eye Disease: Understanding Graves' Ophthalmopathy", which was written by Elaine Moore. Anyone with thyroid eye disease definitely needs to read this book.

Chapter Summary

- Thyroid Eye Disease, also known as Graves' ophthalmopathy, involves the same antibodies which attack the thyroid gland, as these antibodies can also attack the tissues of the eyes.
- Although this condition usually self-resolves, sometimes conventional medical treatment is necessary to help manage the symptoms.
- If someone has Graves' Disease and is following a natural treatment protocol, if this is successful in restoring their health back to normal then in most cases it will prevent thyroid eye disease from developing.
- For someone who already has thyroid eye disease, natural treatment methods can still usually help.

For more information on these and other natural thyroid health topics, visit www.GravesDiseaseBook.com

CHAPTER 21

Natural Treatment Methods During Pregnancy & Lactation

FOR THOSE WOMEN with hyperthyroidism or Graves' Disease who are either pregnant or breastfeeding, there are numerous risks associated with the different hyperthyroid treatment options typically recommended by most endocrinologists. What I plan on doing here is discussing the risks of these conventional treatment methods, and then I will talk about holistic treatment options for pregnant and lactating women. This way you can use this information in order to make an informed decision as to which treatment you would like to receive.

The Conventional Hyperthyroid Treatment Options:

The most common hyperthyroid treatment recommended by endocrinologists and other types of medical doctors for pregnant and lactating women is antithyroid drugs. Methimazole and PTU are two of the most common drugs prescribed, and they can usually do a pretty good job in managing the symptoms of hyperthyroidism. However, there are potential risks to the baby when taking antithyroid drugs. But the risk of untreated hyperthyroidism is usually greater than taking the antithyroid drugs, which is why most endocrinologists usually recommend the latter option.

For those women with hyperthyroidism or Graves' Disease who are pregnant or breastfeeding who don't respond well to antithyroid drugs, the next step usually would be for them to receive thyroid surgery. This procedure is rarely performed on pregnant and lactating women, and is usually reserved for those women with severe symptoms who don't respond well to antithyroid drugs. Since thyroid surgery comes with many risks, most medical doctors will try to avoid this procedure if at all possible.

Radioactive Iodine Therapy IS NOT Recommended For Pregnant Or Lactating Women

This treatment has the potential to obliterate the thyroid gland of the fetus, and as a result, it is not recommended by endocrinologists to women who are pregnant or breastfeeding. This should give you a good idea as to how harsh of a treatment method this is, as you want to be cautious with any treatment that has the word "radioactive" in it. So as I've mentioned already in this book, even in people who aren't pregnant or lactating, radioactive iodine shouldn't be the first treatment option, yet many doctors do in fact recommend this to their "non-pregnant" patients as the primary treatment option.

Natural Treatment Methods:

Another treatment option for women with hyperthyroidism or Graves' Disease who are either pregnant or breastfeeding is to use natural treatment methods to help manage their symptoms. And as I've discussed throughout this book, many times such a protocol can also restore the person's health back to normal. This obviously presents a more appealing option than taking prescription drugs or receiving surgery, and as a result, many pregnant and lactating women are beginning to choose natural treatment methods.

But are natural treatment methods safe for pregnant and lactating women? Under the guidance of a competent natural endocrine doctor, natural treatment methods for pregnant and lactating women with a hyperthyroid condition can be a very safe option. However, there are certain herbs that are contraindicated for pregnancy and lactation, which is yet another reason why it's extremely risky to self treat your condition. A good holistic doctor who focuses on endocrine disorders will be able to determine which supplements and herbs are safe to take while pregnant or breastfeeding, and which ones should be avoided.

This of course doesn't mean that you should stop taking antithyroid medication if you decide to begin a natural treatment protocol. You probably should continue taking any medication you're currently taking, but at the same time might want to consider consulting with a holistic doctor. Then if it's determined that a natural treatment protocol can benefit you, you can either continue taking the antithyroid drugs at the same time, or can wean off of them under the guidance of your medical doctor. In this situation we're obviously not only talking about your health, but also the health of your baby. In fact, many women will choose to remain on the antithyroid medication and follow the natural treatment protocol for the duration of their pregnancy.

The Reason Why Natural Treatment Methods Are So Effective In Pregnant Women

The reason why natural treatment methods are so effective has to do with everything I've spoken about so far in this book. As you know by now, natural treatment methods get to the underlying cause of the condition, rather than just manage the symptoms. While symptom management is important for someone who has severe hyperthyroid symptoms, conventional medical treatment does nothing for the actual cause of hyperthyroidism and Graves' Disease. While taking antithyroid drugs may be necessary to manage the symptoms, in most cases they should be taken on a temporary basis.

On the other hand, you already know that the primary goal of a competent holistic doctor is to determine the actual cause of the condition. This way the holistic doctor can come up with a natural treatment plan to help the pregnant or lactating woman restore her health back to normal. Once again, there are certain restrictions for women who are pregnant or breastfeeding, which is why it's important to consult with an expert, rather than try self-treating your condition.

Which Nutritional Supplements And Herbs Are Dangerous For Pregnant Women?

If you visit your local health food store and look at the supplements and herbs on the shelves, many of them will contain wording which suggests women who are pregnant or lactating need to be cautious when consuming such products. What you need to understand is that many of the nutritional supplements and herbal remedies which have warnings aimed towards pregnant and lactating women aren't necessarily unsafe. With regards to whole food nutritional supplements, there usually is minimal risk when it comes to giving them to a pregnant woman. In fact, it is essential that pregnant women take high quality prenatal vitamins. And since many pregnant women don't eat healthy, taking some additional nutritional supplements is also a good idea (Vitamin D, trace minerals, etc.).

It's a different story with herbs. While many herbs are safe for pregnant women to take, some can also be harmful. To no surprise, no clinical research studies have been done to evaluate the side effects of herbs on pregnant and lactating women (at least none that I'm aware of). This shouldn't be surprising as I know I wouldn't have wanted my wife to participate in such a study when she was pregnant or while she was breastfeeding our children. But this doesn't mean that all herbs are risky for pregnant women to take.

For example, one of the companies I use with regards to nutritional supplementation and herbs is Standard Process, which provides both whole food supplements and herbal remedies. Once again, I wouldn't hesitate to give a pregnant woman most of the whole food supplements available, but there are some herbs I would be cautious about giving, and others which under no circumstances would I give. For example, let's take a look at the "cautions" for the herb Echinacea as listed on the Standard Process packaging:

> *"Not to be used during pregnancy and lactation unless otherwise directed by a qualified health care professional."*

Now let's take a look at the wording for Bugleweed, which is an herb I frequently recommend for people with hyperthyroidism and Graves' Disease (and one that I personally took as part of my natural treatment protocol):

> *"Contraindicated in pregnancy and lactation. Contraindicated in hypothyroidism and enlargement of the thyroid without functional disorder".*

While both of these herbs issue warnings to pregnant and lactating women, you can see the difference between the two warnings. Echinacea warns that it shouldn't be used during pregnancy UNLESS otherwise directed by a qualified healthcare professional. This means they are essentially putting this verbiage down to protect themselves from litigation, but in some cases Echinacea can be taken by pregnant or lactating women while under the guidance of a competent healthcare professional. On the other hand, Bugleweed is clearly contraindicated in pregnancy and lactation, and therefore should not be taken by a pregnant woman under any set of circumstances.

I frequently mention in this book, as well as the articles and posts on my website, how people with hyperthyroidism and Graves' Disease shouldn't self-treat their condition, and this obviously is even more important for pregnant women who have a hyperthyroid condition. And for those who think nutritional supplements and herbs are completely safe because they are "natural", hopefully I've convinced you that this isn't true, and that some herbs can be harmful. This isn't only true with regards to pregnant women, but with anyone, and is especially true when people mix herbs, or combine certain herbs with medication they are taking. This is yet another good reason to consult with a competent natural endocrine doctor.

Combining Different Hyperthyroid Treatment Options During Pregnancy

I of course have dedicated an entire chapter to this, as the downside of natural treatment methods is that it can take a few weeks before they begin to effectively manage the symptoms. As a result, a woman who is pregnant or breastfeeding might want to consider taking the antithyroid drugs on a temporary basis, and at the same time begin a natural treatment protocol under the guidance of a competent holistic doctor. Then after a few months she can choose to wean off the prescription drugs (under the supervision of a competent medical doctor), and continue with the natural treatment protocol. Of course as I mentioned earlier she can instead choose to continue taking the antithyroid medication throughout her pregnancy, and then after she gives birth wean off. Ultimately it's her decision to make, and I have no problem with someone wanting to continue taking the antithyroid medication at the same time they are following a natural treatment protocol.

Using Natural Hyperthyroid Treatment Methods BEFORE Pregnancy

The ideal situation would be to begin using natural treatment methods before becoming pregnant. If you are already pregnant or breastfeeding then you can still of course benefit from a natural treatment protocol. But if you have hyperthyroidism or Graves' Disease and you're not currently pregnant or breastfeeding, then following a natural treatment protocol not only can potentially restore your health back to normal, but it will create a very healthy environment for the baby.

In fact, I think that any woman who is thinking of getting pregnant should incorporate some type of natural treatment protocol not only to optimize her own health, but to also improve the chances of having a healthy baby as well. Without question it isn't easy to follow through with such a protocol, but the benefits make it well worth it, especially when we're talking about the long term health of you and your baby.

Following The Factors Of Health Is Essential To A Healthy Pregnancy

Other than being cautious about taking certain herbs, a pregnant woman can follow most of the other components of a natural treatment protocol. Of course just like anyone else looking to restore their health back to normal, it will be essential for them to make certain changes in their lifestyle, as just taking nutritional supplements and/or herbs alone won't cure someone's hyperthyroid condition. So anyone who is pregnant will want to eat well, obtain quality sleep, do a good job of managing their stress, get some regular exercise, minimize their exposure to environmental toxins, etc. Of course this should be the case for any pregnant woman, and not just someone who has a hyperthyroid condition.

In summary, being pregnant shouldn't prevent someone from following a natural treatment protocol, although there may be some modifications as to which supplements and/or herbs they can take. This might affect the recovery process to some extent, but overall following such a protocol will still greatly benefit the health of both the mother and baby.

Chapter Summary

- For those women with hyperthyroidism or Graves' Disease who are either pregnant or breastfeeding, there are numerous risks associated with the different hyperthyroid treatment options typically recommended by most endocrinologists.

- Because natural treatment options can potentially restore someone's health back to normal, many pregnant and lactating women with hyperthyroid conditions are beginning to choose natural treatment methods.

- Many of the nutritional supplements and herbal remedies which have warnings aimed towards pregnant and lactating women aren't necessarily unsafe, as you need to read the warnings carefully.

- If you have hyperthyroidism or Graves' Disease and you're not currently pregnant or breastfeeding, but are thinking about becoming pregnant, then following a natural treatment protocol not only can potentially restore your health back to normal, but it will create a very healthy environment for the baby.

For more information on these and other natural thyroid health topics, visit www.GravesDiseaseBook.com

CHAPTER 22

Thyroid Storm & Natural Hyperthyroid Treatment Methods

A SMALL PERCENTAGE of people with hyperthyroidism develop a severe condition known as thyroid storm. Even though this condition doesn't affect too many people with hyperthyroidism, those who are affected by thyroid storm need to get this addressed immediately. This condition is an emergency situation, and conventional medical treatment is required.

With that being said, do natural hyperthyroid treatment methods play any role in helping people with thyroid storm? Before I answer this, let's look at some of the common symptoms of this condition. People who have thyroid storm may experience an increased heart rate exceeding 200 beats per minute. They may also experience palpitations, an increase in blood pressure, as well as chest pain and/or a shortness of breath. So it's easy to understand why this is considered to be an emergency situation, and why anyone with thyroid storm needs to see a medical doctor immediately.

Managing The Symptoms Of Thyroid Storm

Due to the severity of the symptoms, usually a combination of different prescription drugs is used to manage the symptoms of thyroid storm. Some of the common drugs recommended to people with this condition include beta blockers, antithyroid drugs, and can also include a blockade iodine drug. Sometimes an infection can be causing or contributing to thyroid storm, and when this is the case this obviously needs to be addressed.

As for using natural treatment methods, you might wonder whether someone with thyroid storm can take certain nutritional supplements or herbs to help manage their symptoms. Even though there are some herbs which can help manage the symptoms of hyperthyroidism, such as Bugleweed and Motherwort, these herbs will usually take some time to "kick in". And when someone has a pulse exceeding 200 beats per minute or has difficulty breathing, they obviously don't have time to wait for natural treatment methods to take effect.

Can Natural Treatment Methods Trigger Thyroid Storm?

I've had some people ask whether beginning a natural treatment protocol can trigger an episode of thyroid storm. In my experience this has never happened, and I honestly have never heard of someone developing thyroid storm due to taking a specific nutritional supplement or herb. The one possible exception is if someone takes large dosages of iodine without any proper testing. Even in this case it's rare, as while I recommend that people begin supplementing with low dosages of iodine (once a deficiency is confirmed), I know some holistic doctors will start patients on 25 to 50 mg of iodine immediately, and some even do this without any testing. Once again, it all comes down to risks vs. benefits, and just like someone might develop thyroid storm while taking antithyroid medication or after receiving radioactive iodine, I guess there is always the chance that they can develop this condition while following a natural treatment protocol as well. But once again, it's something I personally haven't experienced with my patients, and I don't know of anyone else who had thyroid storm triggered due to following a natural treatment protocol.

Preventing Thyroid Storm From Coming Back

Although someone shouldn't use natural treatment methods to manage the symptoms of thyroid storm, after conventional medical treatment methods are used to control the symptoms, then one can use natural treatment methods to attempt to restore the person's health back to normal, and prevent thyroid storm from reoccurring. So at this point one can take Bugleweed, Motherwort, and other nutritional supplements and/or herbs. Of course just taking supplements and herbs alone won't restore your health back to normal, and as a result it's always wise to consult with a competent holistic doctor, rather than self-treat your own condition (as I've already stated numerous times in this book). After all, while many people don't want to take antithyroid drugs continuously, you also shouldn't need to take Bugleweed or any other herb on a permanent basis. The goal should be to get to the underlying cause of the condition if at all possible, and restore your health so you won't need to depend on any medication or herbs.

So for anyone with thyroid storm who has a "natural mindset", it's important to seek immediate medical attention. Then once you have the symptoms under control you can begin a natural treatment protocol to get to the underlying cause of the hyperthyroid condition, and this in turn should help prevent having a future incidence of this condition.

Chapter Summary

- A small percentage of people with hyperthyroidism develop a severe condition known as thyroid storm, which is an emergency situation, and immediate conventional medical treatment is required.
- Due to the severity of the symptoms, usually a combination of different prescription drugs is used to manage the symptoms of thyroid storm.
- Even though there are some herbs which can help manage the symptoms of hyperthyroidism, these herbs will take some time to "kick in". And when someone has a pulse exceeding 200 beats per minute or has difficulty breathing, they obviously don't have time to wait for natural treatment methods to take effect.
- After conventional medical treatment methods is used to control thyroid storm, then one can use natural treatment methods to attempt to restore the person's health back to normal, and prevent thyroid storm from reoccurring.

For more information on these and other natural thyroid health topics, visit www.GravesDiseaseBook.com

CHAPTER 23

5 Reasons Why You Shouldn't Self-Treat Your Hyperthyroid Condition

AFTER OUR INITIAL consultation and listening to my recommendations, Keesha figured that she could correct her hyperthyroid condition on her own. She went ahead and changed her diet, purchased some supplements and herbs, and created her own natural treatment protocol. At first she actually began feeling better, as the Bugleweed and Motherwort she was taking helped to improve her symptoms. But when she received her follow-up blood tests two months later the lab values had worsened. She decided to continue self-treating her condition, and after a couple of months passed by the lab values actually improved. She was ecstatic, and since she was feeling much better she decided to wean herself off of the antithyroid medication she was taking.

She had completely weaned herself off the medication, but a few months later she began experiencing some palpitations again, and when she had more follow-up blood tests they had worsened. At this point Keesha wasn't sure what she should do. Should she take the antithyroid medication again? Or should she try taking different supplements and herbs? She finally decided to stop self-treating her condition, as I received an email from her stating that she was ready to follow my recommendations. She did have to begin taking the antithyroid medication again temporarily, but shortly after beginning a natural treatment protocol she began to wean herself off of them (her own decision of course), and she continuously got better, as her symptoms resolved and her blood tests eventually normalized.

Many people with hyperthyroidism and Graves' Disease don't want to cover up their symptoms by taking antithyroid drugs, and most people want to avoid receiving radioactive iodine therapy if at all possible. This is great, as these people realize there is an underlying cause behind their problem, and they want to attempt treating their condition naturally. Chances are this is why you are reading this book. Of course some people do need to take antithyroid drugs, and some people do need to receive radioactive iodine therapy. But as I've mentioned already, many people with hyperthyroidism and Graves' Disease can restore their health back to normal, and many of these people think they can do so on their own. As a result, they gather as much information as they can through reading books and surfing the internet, and then put together their own natural treatment protocol.

Sometimes people will see positive changes in their symptoms when self-treating their hyperthyroid condition. On the other hand, many people won't see much of a difference. Either way, most people who attempt to self-treat their condition aren't able to successfully restore their health back to normal. So I decided to dedicate this chapter to those people who are looking to take a natural approach, but are thinking about self-treating their condition.

What I'm going to do here is list five reasons why you shouldn't self-treat your condition. This is true whether you have primary hyperthyroidism, or an autoimmune disorder such as Graves' Disease.

Reason #1: There are risks when self-treating your condition. Even when using natural supplements and herbs, there are always risks involved. Most people don't have a strong knowledge of these supplements and herbs, and many assume that because they are natural there is no risk involved. While the risk might be minimal, it still exists. Plus, just abruptly stopping any antithyroid medication you may be taking and replacing these prescription drugs with nutritional supplements and herbs makes it even more risky.

Reason #2: You can't trust everything you read. Once again, many people come up with a natural treatment protocol based on what they read in a book, or viewed on the internet. Heck, some people try to piece the information I provide on my website to develop their own natural treatment protocol. Of course different people will need to take different supplements and herbs, and will also require different dosages. As a result, it's extremely difficult to come up with a treatment plan which will work based on the information you read on my website, this book, or anywhere else.

And much of the information on "natural cures" put out there is by people who don't have much experience with this. Many aren't even healthcare professionals. This doesn't mean there aren't people who are very knowledgeable about natural treatments. You just need to be extremely careful about any information you read about, and especially on the internet.

Reason #3: The body is extremely complex. Although it would be great if one could restore their health back to normal simply by eating well and taking some supplements and herbs, it unfortunately is not this easy. The body is way too complex to restore its health back to normal just by taking supplements and herbs, eating well, etc. Obviously eating well and taking supplements and/or herbs is very important to restore one's health back to normal. But doing this alone won't cure your condition, even though it might allow you to feel better initially. But if you're looking to completely restore your health back to normal, just remember that the body is very complex, and because of this it is highly unlikely you will receive optimal results by self-treating your condition.

Reason #4: It probably will cost you more money in the long run. Many people choose to self-treat their condition because they figure they will save money by taking this approach. After all, they won't need to pay a doctor for an initial consultation or any follow-up visits, and they also will be able to price-shop for any supplements or herbs they take, etc. However, after they realize they aren't going to receive optimal results they will frequently end up consulting with a holistic doctor anyway. So while you might save money initially, in the end it almost always will cost you more money when trying to self-treat your condition.

Reason #5: You most likely won't receive optimal results. This obviously relates to the previous four reasons I just spoke about, as for all of the reasons I have mentioned, it is unlikely you will receive optimal results by self-treating your condition naturally. I do get some emails occasionally from people stating they self-treated their condition and felt much better after doing this. And as I've mentioned, some people will feel better when self-treating their condition. On the other hand, many people don't feel much of a difference at all. But even those people who do feel better when self-treating their condition most likely won't fully restore their health back to normal.

In summary, while it might seem easy enough to self-treat your condition, the truth is that for the reasons I've mentioned above, most people don't receive optimal results when taking this approach. This is why I dedicate a chapter in this book on consulting with a natural endocrine doctor, as anyone who is really serious about restoring their health back to normal really should speak with an expert. While there still isn't any guarantee by taking this approach, you stand a much better chance of restoring your health back to normal than if you were to attempt this on your own.

Chapter Summary

- Sometimes people will see positive changes in their symptoms when self-treating their hyperthyroid condition. But most people who attempt to self-treat their condition aren't able to successfully restore their health back to normal.
- Most people don't have a strong knowledge of these supplements and herbs, and many assume that because they are natural there is no risk involved. While the risk might be minimal, it still exists.
- Different people will need to take different supplements and herbs, and will also require different dosages. As a result, it's extremely difficult to come up with a treatment plan which will work based on the information you read on my website, this book, or anywhere else.
- While you might save money initially by self-treating your condition, in the end it almost always will cost you more money when taking this approach.

For more information on these and other natural thyroid health topics, visit www.GravesDiseaseBook.com

CHAPTER 24

Natural Treatment Methods Really Don't Cure Anything

EVEN THOUGH I do mention the word "cure" at times in this book, as well as on my website, the truth is that natural treatment methods really don't cure anything, as it's the person's body which needs to take all of the credit. I'll explain more about this shortly, but before I do this I want to remind you that in the chapter where I discussed the difference between a cure and a remission I admitted that I honestly don't know whether anybody with hyperthyroidism and Graves' Disease who follows a natural treatment protocol can be permanently cured. And as I also discussed, I think that most people would be fine knowing that their condition can't be completely cured, as long as they were able to maintain a good state of health and avoid taking antithyroid drugs or receive radioactive iodine therapy.

After all, the overall goal is to get you to the point where you are able to visit an endocrinologist, or any medical doctor for that matter, and test completely negative for a hyperthyroid condition. In other words, after following a natural treatment protocol, the goal is that if you were to visit an endocrinologist and if you got tested for a hyperthyroid condition, that EVERY test you received would be negative. Of course one can't rely on tests alone, which is why it's really hard to tell whether someone is ever truly cured or not. This is why I usually use the words "restoring one's health back to normal", rather than "curing your condition", although every now and then I do use the word "cure".

What The Real Goal Of A Natural Treatment Protocol Is:

In any case, when I recommend a natural treatment protocol to a patient, I am telling them to do things which will assist their body in the healing process. Many other healthcare professionals take the same approach. For example, I have a chiropractic degree, and when I had my chiropractic practice and saw people with neck pain, back pain, and other similar conditions, the goal wasn't necessarily to "cure" the back pain condition. In fact, chiropractors aren't trained to cure anything in chiropractic school, as they are taught to deal with spinal subluxations, which are misalignments in the spine which cause nerve interference. This in turn can lead to conditions such as neck pain, back pain, but it can also lead to other health issues as well.

So when someone who is experiencing back pain visits a chiropractor, obviously the chiropractor will want to try relieving the person's pain. But although this is the main reason the person decided to schedule an appointment in the first place, the chiropractor's primary goal isn't to provide pain relief, but is to determine whether there is a spinal subluxation which is causing or contributing to the person's pain, and then correct this spinal subluxation. While correcting the subluxation will frequently eliminate the person's back pain, one needs to also remember that the nerves of the spine supply every organ and tissue in the body. As a result, it's possible that this nerve interference can not only cause back pain, but can lead to other health issues. For example, if the nerve that is being affected is supplying the kidney, then this in turn can cause kidney problems. If there is a spinal subluxation which is affecting the nerve supplying the thyroid gland, then this actually can cause or contribute to a thyroid condition as well.

How Does This Relate To Following A Natural Hyperthyroid Treatment Protocol?

My point here is not to convince you to see a chiropractor, but instead is to reveal to you how most holistic doctors are interested in helping the individual achieve optimal health by giving the body what it needs to self-heal. So when someone goes to a chiropractor with neck or back pain, a good chiropractor will focus on the patient's desires, which is to get relief from their pain. But they will also try to help them achieve optimal spinal health. Similarly, when someone comes to me with hyperthyroidism or Graves' Disease, or any other endocrine disorder, my goal is not to treat and cure the condition, but to give the person what they need to help their body achieve optimal endocrine health (as well as optimal digestive health, hormonal health, etc.).

So when I tell someone to eat well, get sufficient sleep, do a better job of managing their stress, and to take certain nutritional supplements and/ or herbs, I don't do this in order to "cure" their condition. I do this in order to help them restore their health back to normal. Some people think the nutritional supplements and/or herbs they take are used to cure their condition, but these supplements and/or herbs are recommended to assist the compromised body. For example, someone who has severe adrenal fatigue might be able to restore their health by modifying certain lifestyle factors. However, certain supplements and herbs can usually help to assist in the recovery process. The same concept applies with addressing the compromised immune system, as I frequently recommend certain supplements and herbs to help with this.

But as I've mentioned before, if someone is successful in restoring their health back to normal but then begins eating junk food again, neglects their sleep, etc., there is an excellent chance that over time they will suffer a relapse. Or perhaps they won't develop a hyperthyroid condition again, but instead will develop a different condition. Either way, any good holistic doctor won't only try to help a person achieve optimal health, but will also give the person the information and the guidance they need to maintain their health.

The Dentistry Model Provides A Good Example Of Preventative Maintenance

If you want to look at a good model of preventative maintenance, then look no further than your local dentist. Most dentists will not only fill cavities, extract teeth, and perform other dental procedures, but they will also teach the patient how they can maintain healthy teeth. This of course involves brushing one's teeth two or three times each day, flossing daily, and visiting your dentist twice each year for regular checkups and cleanings. However, if someone restores their dental health, but stops brushing their teeth, or perhaps only brushes their teeth every now and then, doesn't floss, and doesn't go to the dentist regularly, then there is a good chance that over time they will develop dental problems.

As difficult as it is to follow a natural treatment protocol and restore one's health back to normal, it's also challenging to maintain one's health. But as I frequently tell people, it's not necessary to live a perfect lifestyle in order to maintain your health. If you eat some junk food every now and then, get stressed out once in awhile, and get only five or six hours of quality sleep once or twice each month, then this most likely won't cause a relapse to occur. If your body is healthy and strong, then it will do a great job of adapting to "acute" stress situations. It's the chronic stress, or frequent bad habits your body can't deal with.

In summary, the goal of this book, as well as my website, isn't to provide you with information to help cure your hyperthyroid condition. And when someone chooses me as their healthcare provider and I consult with them, I'm also not trying to cure anything. I'm just giving them the information and tools necessary for them to achieve optimal health. So for those people who get their health restored back to normal due to my advice, don't thank me, but instead thank your wonderful self-healing body.

Chapter Summary

- Even though I do mention the word "cure" at times in this book, the truth is that natural treatment methods really don't cure anything, as it's the person's body which needs to take all of the credit.
- When I recommend a natural treatment protocol to a patient, I am telling them to do things which will assist their body in the healing process.
- Some people think the nutritional supplements and herbs they take are used to cure their condition, but they are recommended to assist the compromised body.
- As difficult as it is to follow a natural treatment protocol and restore one's health back to normal, it's also challenging to maintain one's health.

For more information on these and other natural thyroid health topics, visit www.GravesDiseaseBook.com

The Keys To Maintaining Your Health After Following A Natural Treatment Protocol

FOR THOSE PEOPLE who have restored their health back to normal naturally, the obvious goal is to maintain their health. Doing this is definitely much easier than restoring one's health back to normal. However, it still can be a challenge for people to maintain their health, and thus prevent a relapse from occurring.

As you know, in order to restore your health from a hyperthyroid condition, it is necessary to eat well, get sufficient sleep, manage your stress, minimize your exposure to environmental toxins, take certain nutritional supplements and/or herbs, etc. Although one usually doesn't need to take such extreme measures when maintaining a state of wellness, they still need to take responsibility for their health.

The Two Most Difficult Lifestyle Factors To Manage

After restoring one's health back to normal, the two most difficult life-style factors to keep up with are eating well and doing a good job of managing stress. With regards to eating well, it's important to understand that you don't need to eat a perfect diet. When initially following a natural treatment protocol one should try to eat only whole foods for the first 30 to 90 days, and sometimes longer than this. As I mentioned in an earlier chapter, avoiding common allergens such as gluten and dairy is also recommended.

After one has restored their health back to normal, it's still important to eat mostly whole foods and minimize the amount of refined foods and sugars. But this doesn't mean that someone can't eat some "bad" foods every now and then. For example, I'll admit that I don't eat a perfect diet. While I eat well most of the time, a few times each week I will eat foods that are considered to be unhealthy. For example, on a good night of going out my family and I will go to the local health food store, and I'll either have a turkey sandwich or wrap, which includes free range turkey, and yes, some type of bread. Sometimes I'll have a free range hamburger with organic fries. While this is definitely healthier than a burger and greasy fries you would purchase at a fast food restaurant, it still isn't considered to be too healthy.

But sometimes I'll admittedly eat worse than this, as every now and then my family and I will go out for pizza at a local pizza place, or we'll get some dessert (chocolate cake, ice cream, etc.). Of course this isn't what I do on a regular basis, as once again, I do eat healthy most of the time. And of course when I initially followed a natural treatment protocol I didn't eat any of these "bad" foods, although I still wasn't 100% perfect, as I did have some Standard Process protein bars a few times each week, when I probably should have had an extra serving of vegetables instead. But otherwise I ate pretty well. Although I'm always trying to maintain a state of wellness, I'd be lying if I told you that I didn't go out occasionally and eat foods that aren't considered to be healthy. For most people who have already restored their health back to normal, eating some junk food every now and then isn't too big of a deal.

Of course there are exceptions to this. I've mentioned earlier in this book that someone who has celiac disease shouldn't eat gluten-based foods every now and then. On the other hand, some doctors tell all of their patients with hyperthyroidism and Graves' Disease that they need to permanently avoid gluten-based foods. I don't agree with this train of thought, although perhaps my opinion will change in the future.

Try Not To Get Stressed Out

In addition to maintaining a healthy diet, it's also important to continue doing a good job of managing your stress. Just as is the case with eating healthy, if you get stressed out every now and then it probably won't lead to a relapse. On the other hand, if you let stress get the best of you frequently then there is a good chance you will become symptomatic again.

Some of my patients ask me what stress management techniques they should use. I personally never used yoga or meditation as a stress management technique, although these both can be effective methods of dealing with stress. To be honest, just eating well, exercising regularly, and being aware of the impact stress can have on my health did wonders when it came to managing the stress in my life. When I was first diagnosed with Graves' Disease I did take Eleuthero to help with the stress response as well. But I didn't incorporate any special technique in order to better manage my stress.

Don't forget to check out the 12 stress management strategies I listed in an earlier chapter. You also might want to check out the website www.

heartmath.com, which involves using biofeedback and emWave technologies to help people better deal with stress. As it states on the website, the emWave helps "you learn to control your physiology through breathing along with your heart rhythms and focusing on positive emotions". This might be a good option for someone who deals with a great amount of stress on a regular basis.

Which Nutritional Supplements Should You Take To Maintain Your Health?

After someone restores their health they won't need to take as many supplements as they were taking while following the natural treatment protocol. In most cases they will just need to take some basic whole food supplements. Here are some of the supplements I currently take on a regular basis for wellness purposes:

1. **Whole food multivitamin supplement.** I feel that just about everyone should take a whole food multivitamin supplement, as no matter how well you eat, it is extremely difficult to get all of the nutrients you need from eating. Most multivitamin supplements sold on the market are synthetic and are of low quality, and so I do recommend taking a whole food supplement.

2. **Trace Minerals.** It also is difficult to get all of the minerals from the food you eat, which is why I take a trace minerals supplement daily.

3. **Iodine.** I personally take 12mg of iodine daily. This seems to work well for me, as the last time I obtained an iodine loading test it was within normal limits. Plus, according to Dr. Guy Abraham, who has done a huge amount of research on iodine, at least 13mg of iodine per day is necessary to maintain iodine sufficiency.[34]

4. **Omega 3 fatty acids.** Most people can also benefit from taking omega 3 fatty acids daily. Once again, it's important not to consume too many omega 3 fatty acids, and you want to check the quality of the supplement by cutting it open to make sure it doesn't have a fishy smell, which means that it's rancid.

5. **Whole food vitamin C complex.** I personally take a whole food Vitamin C supplement each day, which helps to keep the immune system healthy and strong. As I mentioned in an earlier chapter, I recommend not taking synthetic Vitamin C sold in retail stores, which just consists of ascorbic acid.

6. **Digestive enzymes.** Even though someone who has restored their digestive system back to normal shouldn't need to take digestive enzymes, I still take some daily as a "play it safe" mechanism. In other words, I think my digestive system works fine, but I still take a digestive enzyme before each major meal for additional digestive support.

In summary, while restoring your health back to normal can be challenging, it also isn't easy to maintain one's health. However, this doesn't mean that people who have restored their health back to normal need to live a perfect lifestyle and eat a perfect diet. While some people have food allergies and sensitivities which prohibit them from eating certain foods, most people who have already restored their health back to normal can get away with eating some junk food every now and then.

Chapter Summary

- For those people who have restored their health back to normal naturally, maintaining their health can be a challenge.
- After restoring one's health back to normal, for most people the two most difficult lifestyle factors to keep up with are eating well and doing a good job of managing stress.
- Upon restoring one's health back to normal, one doesn't need to eat a perfect diet, but they should still eat mostly whole foods and minimize the refined foods and sugars.
- Maintaining your health won't require as many supplements as when following a natural treatment protocol.

For more information on these and other natural thyroid health topics, visit www.GravesDiseaseBook.com

CHAPTER 26

Consult With A
Natural Endocrine Doctor

WHEN APRIL WAS initially diagnosed with Graves' Disease, she wanted to get to the underlying cause of the problem. So she called a local holistic doctor and scheduled an appointment for a consultation. April wasn't sure if the doctor had much experience with Graves' Disease, but there weren't too many other options, as she preferred to speak with someone face-to-face, and so she figured she would have nothing to lose by giving this doctor a try. The holistic doctor put her on a special diet and advised her to take certain supplements and herbs. April followed the protocol for three months, but she didn't notice much of an improvement with her symptoms.

April attended one of my free webinars, and she then scheduled an appointment to speak with me. I told her that I would love the opportunity to help her, but at the same time I wanted her to give the other holistic doctor a fair chance to help her. After all, while most of my patients notice positive changes quickly, for some people it does take more time. And even though the holistic doctor she was seeing didn't focus on endocrine disorders, I told her she probably should give his protocol a little more time. So she followed his protocol for two more months, still didn't see much of an improvement in her symptoms, or any significant changes with her follow-up blood tests. At that point I agreed to see her, and about five weeks after she began the protocol she began noticing a significant reduction in her symptoms, positive changes in her thyroid blood tests after two months, and about three months later her symptoms were completely gone and her thyroid blood tests were completely normal.

If you have hyperthyroidism or Graves' Disease and want to use natural treatment methods to restore your health back to normal, then you will most likely want to consult with a natural endocrine doctor. However, finding a holistic doctor who focuses on endocrine disorders such as hyperthyroidism or Graves' Disease is no easy task. You of course can choose to speak with a "general" holistic practitioner. However, being someone who personally dealt with Graves' Disease and successfully used natural treatment methods to restore my health back to normal, I strongly recommend speaking with a natural endocrine doctor for optimal results. There are numerous medical doctors, naturopaths, and chiropractors who focus on endocrine disorders such as hyperthyroidism and Graves' Disease.

But how do you find a competent natural endocrine doctor? The best way to find any good doctor is through a referral, as if you know someone who happened to be treated by a natural endocrine doctor and received great results, then this is definitely someone who you will want to contact. Of course most people don't have such a connection, and so they resort to searching for a doctor on their own. This definitely can be a challenge.

What's even more challenging is that some holistic doctors don't want anything to do with hyperthyroidism and Graves' Disease. While most holistic doctors don't have a problem dealing with hypothyroidism and Hashimoto's Thyroiditis, since the symptoms of hyperthyroidism can be life threatening at times, many don't want to take the risk of treating hyperthyroidism and Graves' Disease naturally. And most of those holistic doctors who are willing to help people with hyperthyroid conditions will insist that they take antithyroid drugs to manage the symptoms.

You Don't Need To Speak With Someone Locally

While it would be great if you can find a natural endocrine doctor who practices close to where you live or work so that you can see them in person, the good news is that you usually don't need to speak with a holistic doctor face-to-face in order to receive great results. Assuming you've already been diagnosed with hyperthyroidism or Graves' Disease by an endocrinologist or general medical practitioner, and received a physical examination, then in most cases it's perfectly fine to consult with a doctor remotely over the phone.

In fact, just about all of the patients I personally consult with are through the phone. Since there aren't a lot of holistic doctors that focus on endocrine disorders, most of the people I consult with are from different states, and I also speak with people internationally as well, frequently using Skype. In some cases people were able to visit a local holistic doctor, but they preferred to speak with someone who only dealt with endocrine disorders on a regular basis. Plus, I'm sure it also helped that I personally dealt with my own Graves' Disease condition and followed a natural treatment protocol. Because of this, people with this condition know I could relate with them.

There actually are some nice benefits of speaking with a doctor remotely over the phone. One big advantage is not having to wait in a doctor's office way past your appointment time. Plus, it's nice to speak from the comfort of your own home, or even at work during your lunch break without having to take time off. Plus, you don't have to drive to an office, pay money for gas, deal with rush hour traffic, etc. So convenience is definitely one of the benefits of speaking with a natural endocrine doctor remotely.

Using The Internet To Find A Natural Endocrine Doctor

You of course can also use the internet to search for a holistic doctor who focuses on treating endocrine disorders naturally. You do need to be careful, as there are some doctors who might claim they specialize in endocrine disorders, when the truth is that they accept many other types of cases, and as a result only deal with a handful of hyperthyroid patients on a monthly, or even an annual basis. Let's not forget that hyperthyroidism and Graves' Disease are serious conditions, so you really do want to consult with someone who has a good deal of experience. This doesn't mean you need to consult with a doctor who has seen hundreds or thousands of people with hyperthyroidism and Graves' Disease, but it really is a good idea to see someone who has seen a fair share of people with these conditions.

Getting back to searching on the web, you of course can visit your favorite search engine and type in the words "Natural Endocrine Doctor" or "Natural Thyroid Specialist", and then call some of the doctors listed to determine which one might be a good fit for you. I actually list some websites you can visit in my free guide entitled "The 6 Steps On How To Treat Hyperthyroidism & Graves' Disease Through Natural Methods". If you haven't received your free copy you can get it simply by visiting my website at www.GravesDiseaseBook.com and then just enter your name and email address on the right side of my website.

Speaking With Someone Who Doesn't Focus On Endocrine Disorders

Can you receive results from a holistic doctor who doesn't focus their practice on endocrine disorders? For example, if there is a local naturopathic physician, chiropractor, or holistic medical doctor in your area, is it possible to receive great results under the care of such a doctor? Of course it is possible, as there are holistic doctors who don't focus on endocrine disorders, yet still have some experience helping people with hyperthyroidism and Graves' Disease. The problem is that you don't know who these people are, as it's easy for anyone to tell you they have experience, but it's difficult to know if they are telling the truth.

For example, while numerous chiropractors like myself focus on endocrine disorders, most chiropractors don't focus on such conditions. So if you were to randomly call some of the local chiropractors in your area, there is a good chance that none of them will have much experience helping people with hyperthyroidism and Graves' Disease. There is a better chance that a local naturopathic physician will have had some experience seeing some hyperthyroid patients, but then again, there is also the chance they might not have a lot of experience seeing people with these conditions. In fact, with some holistic doctors you would be their very first person presenting with hyperthyroidism or Graves' Disease.

A good way of finding out whether a holistic doctor focuses on endocrine disorders is to visit their website. If you visit their website and they have hyperthyroidism and Graves' Disease listed, along with many other "general" conditions, then you can easily tell that they don't focus solely on endocrine disorders. Once again, this doesn't mean they don't have experience dealing with hyperthyroid conditions. On the other hand, if their website only focuses on endocrine disorders, or better yet, only thyroid and autoimmune thyroid conditions, AND if they have been in practice for awhile, then you can be confident that they have a good deal of experience seeing people with conditions similar to yours. Then again, there are some doctors who have a "niche" website for different conditions to make it look like they specialize in certain areas. In other words, they might have a separate website for thyroid conditions, another one for digestive disorders, etc.

I'm not going to tell you not to see a "general" holistic practitioner, as in most cases this definitely is a better option than receiving radioactive iodine. But if you have a choice between seeing a general holistic doctor and one who focuses on endocrine disorders, then it's obviously better to see someone who has dealt with a lot of people with hyperthyroidism and Graves' Disease. On the other hand, just because someone focuses on endocrine disorders doesn't mean they have dealt with a large number of people with these conditions, as perhaps they mainly have dealt with hypothyroid conditions, and maybe even focus their practice on other endocrine conditions such as diabetes, women fertility issues, etc.

I Repeat, Self-Treating Your Condition Can Be Risky

One of the reasons why some people with hyperthyroidism and Graves' Disease choose to self-treat their condition is due to the challenge of finding a competent natural endocrine doctor. As I've already discussed in the previous chapter, I'm not a fan of self-treating any thyroid condition naturally, but it's especially unwise to treat hyperthyroidism and Graves' Disease on your own. So once again, please don't self-treat your condition, as in most cases these conditions are too complex to successfully self-treat on your own.

In summary, finding a competent natural endocrine doctor can be a challenge, but if you want to receive optimal results then you really should consider speaking with someone who focuses their practice on endocrine conditions. While it may be tempting to self-treat your condition, for optimal results it's wise to consult with an expert.

Chapter Summary

- If you have hyperthyroidism or Graves' Disease and want to use natural treatment methods to restore your health back to normal, then you will most likely want to consult with a natural endocrine doctor.
- Some holistic doctors don't want anything to do with hyperthyroidism and Graves' Disease, which can make it challenging to find someone to help treat your condition naturally.
- Assuming you've already been diagnosed with hyperthyroidism or Graves' Disease by an endocrinologist or general medical practitioner, and have received a physical examination, then in most cases it's perfectly fine to consult with a doctor remotely over the phone.
- You do need to be careful, as there are some doctors who might claim they specialize in endocrine disorders but who only deal with a handful of hyperthyroid patients on a monthly or annual basis.

For more information on these and other natural thyroid health topics, visit www.GravesDiseaseBook.com

CHAPTER 27

Formulate An Action Plan To Restore Your Health Back To Normal

NOW THAT YOU'RE just about done reading this book, I hope you are convinced that you should at least consider natural treatment methods. Just about everyone with hyperthyroidism and Graves' Disease are told that there is no cure. But you now have the information required to potentially restore your health back to normal, and to help you achieve optimal health in all other areas of your life as well.

What I'd like to do is help you design an action plan to restore your health back to normal. While restoring your health isn't an easy process, and of course isn't possible with everyone who has hyperthyroidism or Graves' Disease, if you're willing to take responsibility for your health then not only can you restore your health back to normal, but you probably will feel much better than you have in years. Much of this chapter will be a summary of what you have read in this book, and in order to help keep you motivated I recommend reviewing this chapter on a weekly basis until you have gone through these steps.

Here are four action steps you can take:

Action Step #1: Have A Natural Attitude. Even if you're not fully convinced that natural treatment methods can restore your health back to normal, this doesn't mean you still can't have a natural mindset. In other words, rather than thinking that drugs and surgery are the solution to every problem, begin to ask yourself what the actual cause of the condition is. With regards to your hyperthyroid disorder, you know this condition didn't develop due to a deficiency of antithyroid drugs or radioactive iodine. Something caused this condition to develop, and therefore for most people the goal should be to find the cause of the condition, rather than just manage the symptoms.

Action Step #2: Modify Certain Lifestyle Factors. Chances are you can make some lifestyle changes which can cause a significant improvement in your condition. For example, if you're currently eating a lot of refined foods and sugars, then make it a goal to incorporate more whole foods into your diet. In fact, you can take it to a different level and completely eliminate any processed foods or sugars for 30 days, drink half your weight in ounces of purified water daily, and then see how you feel. You might not feel too good the first few days after such a dramatic change in your eating habits, but if you stick with it you should feel much better after 30 days.

In addition to eating well, try to get at least seven to eight hours of sleep each night, and more than this would be even better. You also want to try doing a better job of managing your stress. Modifying these lifestyle factors really can do wonders for your health.

Action Step #3: Avoid Radioactive Iodine If At All Possible. Some endocrinologists will tell you that radioactive iodine is the only option. Sometimes this is true, but most of the time, RAI should be the last resort. I honestly can't tell you not to receive radioactive iodine, as this is ultimately a decision you will need to make on your own. But I will tell you to try to avoid it if at all possible. Once again, from a legal standpoint I can't tell anyone not to receive this treatment, but most people who use their common sense should have a good idea whether or not it's truly necessary. While many people who have received radioactive iodine can still benefit from natural treatment methods, those who haven't received this treatment will usually respond much better.

Action Step #4: Consult With A Natural Endocrine Doctor. As I spoke about in great detail in the previous chapter, if you decide to follow a natural treatment protocol, it's best to consult with an expert. You definitely don't want to self-treat your condition. And while you can see a "general" holistic doctor, in my opinion it makes sense to consult with someone who has a great deal of experience dealing with endocrine conditions such as hyperthyroidism and Graves' Disease. This will greatly improve your chances of receiving optimal results.

So these are four action steps you can take to help restore your health back normal. While it's without question a challenge for anyone with hyperthyroidism or Graves' Disease to restore their health back to normal, most people willing to make such a commitment will find it well worth it to follow a natural treatment protocol. The problem is that most people aren't willing to take responsibility for their health, and as a result will choose to live with their condition for the rest of their life, or will receive radioactive iodine and take thyroid hormone on a permanent basis.

With that being said, I'd like to thank you for reading this book. I hope you found the information to be useful, and if so, I really do hope that you will take action. For more information on natural thyroid health, including plenty of articles, videos, blog posts, and to register for my free natural thyroid health webinars, visit www.GravesDiseaseBook.com.

Chapter Summary

- Even if you're not fully convinced that natural treatment methods can restore your health back to normal, this doesn't mean you still can't have a natural mindset.
- Chances are you can make some lifestyle changes which can cause a significant improvement in your condition.
- I can't tell anyone not to receive radioactive iodine, as this is ultimately a decision each individual with hyperthyroidism will need to make on their own. But in most cases it should be the last resort.
- As mentioned in the previous chapter, while you can see a "general" holistic doctor, in my opinion it makes sense to consult with someone who has a great deal of experience dealing with endocrine conditions such as hyperthyroidism and Graves' Disease.

For more information on these and other natural thyroid health topics, visit www.GravesDiseaseBook.com

CHAPTER 28

Your Number One Free Resource Center For Natural Thyroid Health

IF YOU ENJOYED reading this book, I highly recommend visiting my website, which is www.GravesDiseaseBook.com. Many of the topics covered in this book are also on my website, and it also provides many other interesting topics as well. As of writing this book, the following is just some of the free material you can access by visiting this website:

Free 42-Page Guide: On my website I offer a free guide which provides a lot of great information on natural thyroid health. It is called "The 6 Steps On How To Treat Hyperthyroidism and Graves' Disease Through Natural Methods". This guide includes information on how to find a competent holistic doctor who focuses on endocrine disorders. Just to let you know, in order to obtain the free guide I do require people to submit their name and email address, which not only gives you access to this free guide, but will also give you email updates whenever I release a new article, blog post, or have a webinar on natural thyroid health.

This free guide consists of 100% content, and is not a sales pitch for any product or service. I feel it's important to state this, as I know there are some websites which offer "free reports" and other free information, which usually are sales letters in disguise. But once again, there are no catches to obtaining this free guide, and of course you are always welcome to cancel your email subscription at any time.

Weekly Blog Post. Each week I create a new post on my blog which usually relates to natural thyroid health, although every now and then I do talk about something different. Either way, these posts on natural health will frequently provide you with useful information to help you achieve optimal health. Here are just some of the blog post topics I have posted in the past:
- 7 Tips To Help You Have A Healthy Digestive System
- Yes, Taking The Pill Can Affect Your Thyroid Health
- Certain Ingredients Can Be Toxic To Your Thyroid Gland
- The Dangers Of Steroid Medications & How They Affect Thyroid Health
- Restoring Your Health Without Bioidentical Hormones

Dozens Of Articles. I also have an articles page where you can access dozens of different articles. There are plenty of articles on hyperthyroidism and Graves' Disease, plus other articles on natural thyroid health. I have received plenty of emails from people who benefited from these articles, and I'm of course hoping that you will benefit from them too.

Videos. Most of the videos on my website have been created through YouTube. To be honest, most of the content of the videos is similar to the articles on the website, but I realize that some people prefer to watch videos rather than read articles, which is why I have created them. Besides visiting my website to watch these videos you also might want to subscribe to my YouTube channels in order to receive updates on any new videos I release. My primary YouTube channel is NaturalThyroidDoctor, although I have another channel called HyperthyroidismCure. I eventually embed any new YouTube videos I create on my website as well.

Free Webinars. Each month I offer free natural thyroid health webinars. These webinars are usually about 45 minutes long, and I provide some valuable information for people with hypothyroidism, hyperthyroidism, and autoimmune thyroid conditions. The following are some of the webinar topics that have been covered:
- 7 Natural Thyroid Treatment Tips To Restore Your Health Back To Normal
- Natural Treatment Solutions For Hyperthyroidism & Graves' Disease
- Natural Treatment Solutions For Hypothyroidism & Hashimoto's Thyroiditis

Facebook Page: I also have a couple of Facebook pages you might want to check out. One of them is called Natural Solutions For Graves' Disease & Hashimoto's Thyroiditis, which you can become a fan of by visiting www.facebook.com/NaturalThyroidTreatment. Another one is called Graves Disease & Hyperthyroidism: Natural Treatment Solutions, which you can become a fan of by visiting www.facebook.com/NaturalHyperthyroidTreatment.

So if you haven't received enough natural thyroid health information in this book, then please visit my website and sign up to receive my free guide and email updates on natural thyroid health. And if you crave even more information on natural thyroid health then of course you're welcome to become a fan of my Facebook pages and a subscriber of my YouTube Channel.

CHAPTER 29

Questions You May Have About Natural Thyroid Treatment Methods

Question #1: Should Gluten Be Avoided In People With Hyperthyroidism & Graves' Disease?

There is a lot of controversy involving gluten consumption in people with autoimmune disorders such as Graves' Disease. I'm honestly still not convinced that everyone with an autoimmune condition needs to avoid gluten for the rest of their life, unless if they have Celiac Disease. Although I do minimize my consumption of gluten-based foods, I do eat foods with gluten occasionally. And while some healthcare professionals will recommend for people with Graves' Disease to avoid gluten-based foods for at least six months, I only avoided such foods for the first 30 days when I followed a natural treatment protocol. Although I realize that symptoms don't tell the entire story, as long as I'm feeling good, my labs are normal, etc., then I'm not going to personally give up gluten for six months or longer at this point.

With that being said, my feelings about gluten has changed somewhat, and if I had to begin a natural treatment protocol all over again I would probably avoid gluten for the first six months. Currently I still recommend for my patients to avoid gluten for at least 30 days, and most people do respond well when taking this approach. But because some people have gluten sensitivity problems it of course won't hurt for people to avoid gluten longer than this, and will only benefit them.

Question #2: Can Goiter Be Cured In People With Hyperthyroidism & Graves' Disease?

Goiter is a condition that is characterized by an enlargement of the thyroid gland. In people with hyperthyroidism and Graves' Disease it is usually caused by the overproduction of thyroid hormone, although it can also be caused by a malignancy, or an iodine deficiency. The typical goiter treatment consists of treating the hyperthyroid condition through antithyroid drugs or radioactive iodine. In some severe cases surgery is required, especially if the person has an obstruction that is causing difficulty in swallowing and/or breathing.

When goiter is caused by an excess production of thyroid hormone, or an iodine deficiency, then many times it's possible to correct this problem through a natural treatment protocol. When I was initially diagnosed with Graves' Disease I had a small goiter, and at times it caused difficulty swallowing. This resolved when following a natural treatment protocol. Sometimes a larger goiter won't respond well to natural treatment methods. Other times the goiter will decrease, but won't completely be cured.

Question #3: If It Is Determined That I'm Deficient In Iodine, How Much Should I Take?

This is not an easy question to answer. Some holistic doctors will start everybody with 25mg to 50mg of iodine, which in my opinion is too high of a dosage for some people. As I mentioned in the chapter on iodine, I will start my patients on 3mg of iodine, and then will have them slowly increase the dosage. How much they take will depend on how deficient they are. Someone who is mildly deficient might only take 12mg of iodine, and sometimes less than this. On the other hand, someone with a moderate to severe deficiency will need to take higher dosages of iodine. Of course follow-up testing should be done to make sure someone is taking a sufficient amount of iodine.

Question #4: How Do I Find A Competent Natural Endocrine Doctor In My Area?

It can be challenging to find a competent holistic doctor who focuses on endocrine disorders. Remember that there isn't any official natural endocrine doctor license or certification, and as a result it can be difficult to prove whether someone truly focuses their practice on conditions such as hyperthyroidism and Graves' Disease. A good place to start is to call some of the local holistic doctors in your area (chiropractors, naturopathic physicians, holistic medical doctors, etc.) and find out if any of them focus on endocrine disorders.

How do you do this? One thing you can do is visit their website, as if their website lists many different conditions then you know that they don't focus on endocrine disorders. Another thing I would do is call each office and ask the person you speak with the following question: "What are the main 3 conditions the doctor focuses on?" If they answer with "we see all different types of conditions", or if one of their top three conditions isn't hyperthyroid conditions, then you know they don't focus on hyperthyroidism and Graves' Disease.

As I mentioned previously, if you can't find someone locally who focuses on endocrine disorders, then you should consider speaking with someone remotely over the phone. As long as you have already been diagnosed by an endocrinologist then in most cases you don't need to see the holistic doctor in person. But I do understand that many people prefer to speak with someone face to face, and if you put in some time calling different practices in and near where you live, you just might find a local holistic doctor who can help you.

Question #5: Do You Accept New Patient Consultations?

As of writing this book I am accepting a limited number of new patient consultations. For more information, visit the "Consultations" page on my website www.GravesDiseaseBook.com.

Question #6: I Took Bugleweed For My Hyperthyroid Symptoms And It Didn't Work. Can You Explain Why?

Although Bugleweed will help many people with hyperthyroidism and Graves' Disease, there are some people who take it and don't notice much of a change in their symptoms. First of all, remember that it can take a few weeks before beginning to experience a decrease in the hyperthyroid symptoms. In some people it can actually take four to six weeks before noticing a difference, although most people should notice a decrease in their symptoms sooner than this. Also, keep in mind that someone who has severe hyperthyroid symptoms might not be able to have their symptoms managed by taking Bugleweed alone. Some people will need to take Motherwort and/or Lemon Balm, while others will need to take antithyroid medication to manage the symptoms.

Question #7: What Should I Do If I'm Allergic To Antithyroid Medication And Have Severe Symptoms?

I've had a few people tell me they have severe hyperthyroid symptoms and are allergic to antithyroid medication, and therefore will need to receive radioactive iodine. First of all, it is rare that someone is allergic to both PTU and Methimazole. So if someone is allergic to PTU, for example, then they probably can take Methimazole, and vice versa. There are always exceptions, and of course it is important to manage the symptoms. Keep in mind that the main dangers are with the cardiac symptoms, such as the high pulse rate, and if someone is allergic to the antithyroid medication and has severe symptoms, they probably will be able to take a beta blocker to manage the symptoms until the natural treatment methods take effect. It ultimately is up to the patient as to what they decide to do, as my goal is not to talk someone out of receiving radioactive iodine, but is once again to present them with the different options they have so they can make an informed decision, and not feel as if they're being pressured by their endocrinologist to receive radioactive iodine, or any other treatment method.

Question #8: Can Natural Treatment Methods Help People With Subclinical Hyperthyroidism?

Just as is the case with primary hyperthyroidism or Graves' Disease, many people with subclinical hyperthyroidism can be helped naturally. Sometimes it can be more challenging helping these people, mainly because the TSH is the only lab value which is usually positive, and they are experiencing minimal symptoms when first consulting with them. As a result, it could be difficult to tell whether someone is responding to a natural treatment protocol from a symptomatic standpoint. Obviously one shouldn't rely on symptoms alone, but symptoms are still important in monitoring a person's response to a natural treatment protocol. In people with subclinical hyperthyroidism it is even more important to look at other tests such as an Adrenal Stress Index test or hair mineral analysis, so they can clearly see that they have other positive findings, and not just a low TSH.

Question #9: Isn't Iodine Deficiency Rare Since Many People Consume Iodized Salt?

Many sources will claim that iodine deficiency in the United States is rare due to iodized salt. But while iodized salt can usually prevent goiter from occurring, in most cases iodized salt isn't sufficient to prevent or correct an iodine deficiency.[35] Once again, there is a lot of controversy involving iodine, and what I recommend is visiting the library and doing some research on your own, and also reading the book "Iodine, Why I Need It, and Why I Can't Live Without It", by Dr. David Brownstein.

Question #10: Can Iodine Cause The Development Of An Autoimmune Thyroid Disorder?

Some sources say that taking iodine can actually induce hyperthyroidism or Graves' Disease. Perhaps if someone is put on a very high dosage of iodine then this could trigger an autoimmune response, or cause a hyperthyroid condition. But as I've already stated, I personally have taken up to 25 mg of iodine without a problem, and many of my patients with hyperthyroidism and Graves' Disease have taken iodine without any problems as well.

Question #11: Do You Have Any Advice For Picky Eaters When It Comes To Following A Natural Treatment Protocol?

Even though I eat relatively healthy now, I have always considered myself to be a picky eater. I grew up eating cold cereal for breakfast, hamburgers, spaghetti, plenty of canned foods, cookies and cakes, soda and punch, etc. I rarely ate vegetables growing up, and as a result I've never been a vegetable lover. I never ate organic food growing up, never went to a health food store until I went to chiropractic college, and I was always hesitant to try new foods. Even to this day I have the same problem, as while I eat healthy, I don't eat a wide variety of foods.

However, I am a lot better than I was in the past, and the best advice I can give to picky eaters is to slowly start changing your eating habits. If you're living off fast food and hate eating vegetables, I don't expect you to immediately begin eating three to five servings of vegetables each day. If this is the case I would begin with one serving of vegetables per day, and then try to add one additional serving each week. You also might want to look into different types of seasonings to help make the taste of vegetables more appealing.

Question #12: Can Someone Have Both Graves' Disease and Hashimoto's Thyroiditis At The Same Time?

It is possible to have the antibodies for both Graves' Disease and Hashimoto's Thyroiditis at the same time. As a result, a person can fluctuate back and forth between hyperthyroidism and hypothyroidism, although this is rare. Some people who have both antibodies wonder if they can benefit from following a natural treatment protocol, and most people with both types of antibodies are able to benefit from natural treatment methods.

Question #13: How Can One Address A Copper Toxicity Problem?

While many people with hyperthyroidism and Graves' Disease are deficient in copper, some people have a copper toxicity problem. Some of the common symptoms include headaches, fatigue, insomnia, and depression. One thing to keep in mind is that sometimes there is plenty of copper in the person's system, but it is biounavailable. This means that it is not being properly utilized by the body. With a copper deficiency one of course needs to take copper to address this problem. With a copper toxicity problem one needs to take certain supplements such as copper chelators (i.e. molybdenum, Spanish Black Radish), supplements which focus on adrenal health (the adrenals help with copper metabolism), as well as some other supplements.

Question #14: Can Someone With a Toxic Multinodular Goiter Be Helped Through A Natural Treatment Protocol?

Just as the name implies, a multinodular goiter is a goiter which contains multiple nodules. I have had some success helping people with multinodular goiters naturally. However, it does seem like people with this condition don't respond as well when following a natural treatment protocol. I of course still recommend that people with this condition give natural treatment methods a try, especially if radioactive iodine or thyroid surgery is recommended. The worst case scenario is that you don't respond well, and if this happens you can always choose to receive the conventional treatment options. On the other hand, if the natural treatment methods are effective then you of course won't need to have your thyroid gland obliterated through RAI or surgically removed.

Question #15: Can A Vegetarian Receive Good Results When Following A Natural Treatment Protocol?

One of the main challenges to being a vegetarian is trying to consume enough protein. While vegetarians of course won't eat any beef or poultry, some will eat fish, which definitely will make it easier. If you don't eat fish, then obviously you can get protein from sources such as eggs (assuming you're not a vegan), nuts and seeds, lentils, etc. Many vegetarians will get a lot of their protein from soy, but since unfermented soy products can have a negative effect on a person's health, one does need to be careful not to consume too much soy.

Question #16: I Thought Most People With Hyperthyroidism Lose Weight. Why Am I Gaining Weight?

Although most people with hyperthyroidism and Graves' Disease do in fact lose weight, some people with a hyperthyroid condition gain weight. This frequently occurs when taking the antithyroid medication, which of course reduces the excess production of thyroid hormone, and can potentially lead to weight gain. Insulin resistance can also be a factor, as well as a condition such as estrogen dominance. A competent holistic doctor will address these conditions, which is necessary when helping someone restore their health back to normal, and will usually also help with any weight gain problems.

Question #17: Can Taking Bioidentical Hormones Help With Hyperthyroidism and Graves' Disease?

I know there is a "bioidentical craze" going on, where natural progesterone and other bioidentical hormones are being taken for many different conditions. I'm personally not one to recommend bioidentical hormones unless absolutely necessary. And I find that most people don't need to take natural progesterone or other bioidentical hormones, even when a hormone deficiency is present. I'm always interested in finding out the underlying cause of the problem. Of course if someone has received a complete hysterectomy, then they might need to take natural progesterone on a continuous basis. On the other hand, if the progesterone deficiency is due to a communication problem between the hypothalamus and the pituitary gland, then why not fix this problem? So if someone with hyperthyroidism or Graves' Disease has a hormone imbalance, taking bioidentical hormones might help, but if possible I will try to correct the hormone imbalance without giving natural hormones.

Question #18: How Accurate Is A Hair Mineral Analysis Test?

The hair mineral analysis is not a well understood test, and because of this many doctors dismiss the test as being inaccurate. This actually is one of the most valuable tests out there, although I do admit that it can be confusing to the patient (and sometimes to the doctor!). If the hair mineral analysis is done by a good lab then the results should be accurate. For example, some hair analysis labs wash the hair right before analyzing the sample, which will affect some of the minerals. Washing the hair prior to analyzing can wash out the water-soluble elements, which will lead to less accurate results. So you definitely want to choose a lab that doesn't wash the hair prior to analyzing the hair sample.

Question #19: Should One Remove Heavy Metals When Following A Natural Treatment Protocol?

A hair mineral analysis test will help to identify some of the more common heavy metal toxicities, such as aluminum, mercury, and lead. One doesn't necessary have to remove all of the heavy metals in order to restore one's health back to normal. However, this doesn't mean that one shouldn't try to remove, or at least reduce the amount of heavy metals in a person's body. For example, it's very common for people to have high aluminum levels on the hair mineral analysis. While it probably will be impossible to completely eliminate the aluminum from a person's body, this doesn't mean that it can't be lowered. The same can be said with mercury, as if someone has high mercury levels, the goal will be to get the levels as low as possible. With that being said, I usually don't put anyone on a heavy metal detoxification protocol immediately upon starting a natural treatment protocol. What I will typically do is recommend a follow-up hair mineral analysis test after someone has restored their health back to normal. I do this to look at the mineral levels, and at this point if the person still has high levels of heavy metals then I will recommend a heavy metal detoxification. There of course are some things the patient might need to do on their own. For example, if they have high mercury levels due to the fillings in their teeth, then eventually it would be a good idea to get these removed.

Question #20: Can Someone Who Has Already Received Radioactive Iodine Treatment Really Have Their Thyroid Health Restored Back To Normal?

The goal here isn't to offer false hope to people who have already received radioactive iodine treatment. So let me begin by stating that for someone who has already received RAI, it will be much more difficult to restore their health when compared to someone who hasn't received this treatment procedure. On the other hand, some people who have received RAI can restore their thyroid health. This doesn't mean that natural treatment methods will completely reverse the damage caused by the radioactive iodine, but sometimes it can get the thyroid gland to a point where it will produce a sufficient amount of thyroid hormone on its own so that the person doesn't need to take synthetic or natural thyroid hormone on a permanent basis.

Of course there is a decent chance that someone who has received radioactive iodine won't have their thyroid health restored back to normal, and may need to take thyroid hormone continuously. But as I have mentioned many times in this book, radioactive iodine won't do anything to address the cause of hyperthyroidism and Graves' Disease. So even if it's not possible to get the thyroid gland to produce a sufficient amount of thyroid hormone on its own, most of these people still can benefit from natural treatment methods in order to have the health restored of other areas which may be compromised (adrenal glands, immune system, digestive system, etc.).

Question #21: What Do You Think About The Following Holistic Methods With Regards To Treating Hyperthyroid Conditions?

1. **Chiropractic.** Although numerous chiropractors like myself help people with conditions such as hyperthyroidism and Graves' Disease, chiropractic care itself won't provide a cure for this condition. This doesn't mean that chiropractic care can't benefit people with hyperthyroid conditions. While most people perceive chiropractors as being neck and back pain doctors, chiropractic is more than just helping people get relief from their pain. I'm not going to get into detail about chiropractic, but chiropractors deal with subluxations, which essentially are misalignments that affect the nervous system. As you probably know, the nerves supply every organ, tissue, and cell in the body. And so while a subluxation can cause pain, it can definitely do more than this.

For example, if someone has a subluxation affecting the nerves which supply the thyroid gland, then it's possible this can affect one's thyroid health. Can it lead to a hyperthyroid condition? I honestly don't know, but if I had such a subluxation I know that I would want to have it corrected. Similarly, subluxations can affect any other gland or organ in the body. Having one or more subluxations can also affect the immune system as well, which obviously is very important in people with Graves' Disease. So while chiropractic care itself isn't required to restore the health of most people with hyperthyroidism and Graves' Disease, having one or more subluxations can potentially affect someone's recovery, and from an overall health perspective, many people with hyperthyroid conditions can benefit from chiropractic care.

2. **Acupuncture.** Just as is the case with chiropractic, many people can benefit from acupuncture. But receiving acupuncture alone usually won't restore the health of someone who has hyperthyroidism or Graves' Disease. On the other hand, combining acupuncture with changes in lifestyle factors, along with certain supplements and/or herbs will probably be more effective. So both chiropractic care and acupuncture can benefit the health of people with hyperthyroid conditions, and remove some interferences which can potentially prevent someone from having their health restored back to normal. But just receiving chiropractic care or acupuncture alone usually won't be sufficient to restore one's health back to normal.

3. **Homeopathy.** I personally don't know anyone with hyperthyroidism and Graves' Disease who has had their health restored back to normal using homeopathic remedies, but this doesn't mean that homeopathy can't be beneficial. I would definitely give homeopathy a try before receiving radioactive iodine or thyroid surgery. If seeking a healthcare professional who uses homeopathy I would try to work with someone who focuses on thyroid and autoimmune thyroid conditions.

4. **Johnson method.** If you're not familiar with the Johnson method, you can learn more about it by visiting www.iThyroid.com. The website was created by John Johnson, who had a hyperthyroid condition and restored his health naturally, mainly by changing his diet and address-

ing certain nutritional deficiencies. I personally never tried his protocol, and while I don't agree with everything he states on his website, overall there is some great information and I definitely would recommend anyone with hyperthyroidism or Graves' Disease to check it out.

When it comes down to it, I do think there are different ways of accomplishing the same thing. In other words, I'm sure the protocols I recommend to people with hyperthyroidism and Graves' Disease aren't the only effective protocols in restoring one's health back to normal. Different holistic doctors will have different recommendations, and when it comes to avoiding radioactive iodine treatment and preserving the health of your thyroid gland, I think it's worth giving these or other holistic treatment methods a try.

About The Author

DR. ERIC OSANSKY is a licensed healthcare professional who personally restored his health back to normal through natural treatment methods after being diagnosed with Graves' Disease. He has also helped many others with hyperthyroidism and Graves' Disease restore their health naturally.

Dr. Osansky is a chiropractic physician, and although he focused on traditional chiropractic conditions for 7 ½ years, after being diagnosed with Graves' Disease and realizing how well natural treatment methods worked, he began helping other people with hyperthyroid conditions restore their health back to normal.

While Dr. Osansky feels that most people with hyperthyroidism and Graves' Disease should give natural treatment methods a try, he does realize that there is a time and place for conventional medical treatment such as antithyroid medication, and even radioactive iodine in certain situations. And while he of course wants to help everyone with a hyperthyroid condition, Dr. Osansky won't hesitate to refer someone out if he feels as if they are not a good candidate for natural treatment methods.

Dr. Osansky lives in Charlotte, North Carolina with his wife Cindy, and two daughters Marissa and Jaylee.

As of writing this book Dr. Osansky does accept a limited number of new patient consultations each month for people with hyperthyroid conditions looking to restore their health naturally. Those people who are interested in scheduling a consultation with Dr. Osansky should visit his "Consultations" page on his website, www.GravesDiseaseBook.com.

Resources

Books I Recommend:

Adrenal Fatigue: The 21st Century Stress Syndrome by James L. Wilson

The Autoimmune Epidemic by Donna Jackson Nakazawa and Dr. Douglas Kerr

Feeling Fat, Fuzzy, or Frazzled? A 3-Step Program to: Restore Thyroid, Adrenal, and Reproductive Balance, Beat Hormone Havoc, and Feel Better Fast! by Richard Shames and Karilee Shames

Graves' Disease: A Practical Guide by Elaine A. Moore and Lisa Moore

Iodine, Why You Need It, Why You Can't Live Without It by Dr. David Brownstein

Living Well with Graves' Disease and Hyperthyroidism: What Your Doctor Doesn't Tell You...That You Need To Know by Mary J. Shomon

Thyroid Eye Disease: Understanding Graves' Ophthalmopathy by Elaine A. Moore

What Your Doctor May Not Tell You About Menopause: The Breakthrough Book on Natural Hormone Balance by John R. Lee and Virginia Hopkins

Zapped: Why Your Cell Phone Shouldn't Be Your Alarm Clock and 1,268 Ways To Outsmart the Hazards Of Electronic Pollution by Ann Louise Gittleman

Websites I Recommend:

www.NaturalEndocrineSolutions.com
This is my primary website on natural thyroid health, as I have numerous articles, blog posts, and videos on hyperthyroid and hypothyroid conditions, including Graves' Disease and Hashimoto's Thyroiditis.

www.GravesDiseaseBook.com
This website was created specifically for people with hyperthyroidism and Graves' Disease who are looking for a natural treatment solution. It also has numerous articles, videos, etc. I also offer a free guide entitled "The 6 Steps On How To Treat Hyperthyroidism & Graves' Disease Through Natural Methods".

www.elaine-moore.com
This website is from the author of the book "Graves Disease, A Practical Guide", and has some excellent information, including articles, updated blog posts, along with other resources.

www.thyroid.about.com
This is the website of Mary Shomon, and she does a great job of providing up-to-date information on thyroid health.

http://forums.about.com/n/pfx/forum.aspx?webtag=ab-thyroid2
This is a forum called "Ask Elaine Moore", which is for people with hyperthyroidism and Graves' Disease, and is hosted by About.com and moderated by Mary Shomon.

www.livingwithgravesdisease.com/forums/
This is a forum specifically for people with Graves' Disease. This is an excellent site for those looking to communicate with others who have a hyperthyroid condition.

www.dearthyroid.org/tag/graves-disease-blog/
The goal of this website is to "create a community of thyroid patients that feel safe and comfortable writing about their disease."

http://www.aarda.org/
This is the website to the American Autoimmune Related Diseases Association. As stated in their mission statement, "The American Autoimmune Related Diseases Association is dedicated to the eradication of autoimmune diseases and the alleviation of suffering and the socio-economic impact of autoimmunity through fostering and facilitating collaboration in the areas of education, public awareness, research, and patient services in an effective, ethical and efficient manner."

www.ithyroid.com
This website was created by John Johnson, who cured his hyperthyroid condition naturally, primarily by correcting certain nutritional deficiencies. This website contains a lot of interesting information for people with hyperthyroidism and Graves' Disease.

http://webhome.idirect.com/~wolfnowl/thyroid.htm
The website for "Mike's Graves Disease Page", which discusses alternative methods of treatment. The person who created the website (Mike Pedde) was diagnosed with Graves' Disease, and worked with a holistic doctor to restore his health back to normal.

www.drlwilson.com
This is one of my favorite websites on natural health, and while the focus isn't on thyroid and autoimmune thyroid conditions, a lot of the information can benefit people with hyperthyroid conditions.

www.Mercola.com
Although this website doesn't specifically focus on thyroid and autoimmune conditions, this is one of the most well known websites on natural health, and does have a lot of interesting information.

Testing From Companies I Recommend:

> *NOTE: Some of these labs require a licensed healthcare professional to authorize the ordering of these tests*

Blood and Laboratory Testing:
Direct Laboratory Services
4040 Florida St.
Suite 202
Mandeville, LA 70448
www.directlabs.com

Food Allergy Testing:
Genova Diagnostics
63 Zillicoa Street
Asheville, NC 28801

1-800-522-4762
www.gdx.net

Hair Mineral Analysis Testing:
Analytical Research Labs
2225 West Alice Avenue
Phoenix, AZ 85021 USA
1-602-995-1580
www.arltma.com

Iodine Testing
Hakala Research
88# Parfet St.
Suite C
Lakewood, CO 80215
303-763-6242
www.hakalalabs.com

Saliva-based Adrenal and Hormone Testing:
Diagnos-Techs
19110 66th Ave S, Bldg G
Kent, WA 98032 USA
425-251-0596
www.diagnostechs.com

References

1, 2   http://www.nytimes.com/2010/03/24/health/24birth.html

3   Plourde, Elizabeth. Your Guide to Hysterectomy, Ovary Removal, & Hormone Replacement. 2002: 38-39

4   Nakazawa, Donna Jackson. The Autoimmune Epidemic. 2006: 106

5   Nakazawa, Donna Jackson. The Autoimmune Epidemic. 2006: 72

6   Wilson, Dr. James L. Wilson. Adrenal Fatigue, The 21st Century Stress Syndrome. 2010: 270

7   Nakazawa, Donna Jackson. The Autoimmune Epidemic. 2006: 250

8   The relationship of psychological factors to the prognosis of hyperthyroidism in antithyroid drug-treated patients with Graves' disease. By: Fukao, Atsushi; Takamatsu, Junta; Murakami, Yasuhiro; Sakane, Sadaki; Miyauchi, Akira; Kuma, Kanji; Hayashi, Shunichiro; Hanafusa, Toshiaki. Clinical Endocrinology, May2003, Vol. 58 Issue 5, p550-555, 6p

9   http://www.webmd.com/diet/features/why-you-need-more-fiber

10   Influence of physiological dietary selenium supplementation on the natural course of autoimmune thyroiditis. By: Nacamulli, Davide; Mian, Caterina; Petricca, Daniela; Lazzarotto, Francesca; Barollo, Susi; Pozza, Dina; Masiero, Stefano; Faggian, Diego; Plebani, Mario; Girelli, Maria E.; Mantero, Franco; Betterle, Corrado. Clinical Endocrinology, Oct2010, Vol. 73 Issue 4, p535-539, 5p, 1 Black and White Photograph, 1 Chart, 3 Graphs

11   3. Benvenga S, et al. 2001 Usefulness of l-carnitine, a naturally occurring peripheral antagonist of thyroid hormone action, in iatrogenic hyperthyroidism: A randomized, double-blind, placebo-controlled clinical trial. Journal of Clinical Endocrinology & Metabolism 86(8):3579-3594

12   Carcinogenic chromium(VI) induces cross-linking of vitamin C to DNA in vitro and in human lung A549 cells. Quievryn George; Messer Joseph; Zhitkovich Anatoly; Biochemistry 2002 Mar 5; 41 (9): 3156-67

13   Brownstein, Dr. David . Iodine, Why You Need It, Why You Can't Live Without It. 2009: 48

14   Brownstein, Dr. David . Iodine, Why You Need It, Why You Can't Live Without It. 2009: 228

15   Clinical Endocrinology; Sep2009, Vol. 71 Issue 3, p440-445, 6p, 3 Charts, 1 Graph

16   The Effect of Small Doses of Stable Iodine in Patients with Hyperthyroidism.. By: Volpe, Robert; Johnston, MacAllister W.. Annals of Internal Medicine, Apr62, Vol. 56 Issue 4, p577, 13p

17   Brownstein, Dr. David . Iodine, Why You Need It, Why You Can't Live Without It. 2009: 136

18   Nakazawa, Donna Jackson. The Autoimmune Epidemic. 2006: 255

19   Lee, Dr. John R. What Your Doctor May Not Tell You About Menopause. The Breakthrough Book on Natural Hormone Balance. 2004: 62

20   Lee, Dr. John R. What Your Doctor May Not Tell You About Menopause. The Breakthrough Book on Natural Hormone Balance.2004:63

21   http://www.thyroid-info.com/autoimmune/work.htm

22   Nakazawa, Donna Jackson. The Autoimmune Epidemic. 2006: 72

23   Moore, Elaine A. and Moore, Lisa. Graves' Disease, A Practical Guide. 2001: 107

24   Moore, Elaine A. and Moore, Lisa. Graves' Disease, A Practical Guide. 2001: 109

25   What is the role of radioiodine uptake measurement and thyroid scintigraphy in the diagnosis and management of hyperthyroidism? By: Franklyn, Jayne A.. Clinical Endocrinology, Jan2010, Vol. 72 Issue 1, p11-12, 2p

26   http://www.nlm.nih.gov/medlineplus/ency/article/003689.htm

27   Increased long-term cardiovascular morbidity among patients treated with radioactive iodine for hyperthyroidism. By: Metso, Saara; Auvinen, Anssi; Salmi, Jorma; Huhtala, Heini; Jaatinen, Pia. Clinical Endocrinology, Mar2008, Vol. 68 Issue 3, p450-457, 8p, 3 Charts, 2 Graphs

28   TMortality after the Treatment of Hyperthyroidism with Radioactive Iodine. By: Franklyn, J.A.; Maisonneuve, P.; Sheppard, M.C.; Betteridge, J.; Boyle, P.. New England Journal of Medicine, 03/12/98, Vol. 338 Issue 11, p712-718, 1p

29   Choice of Therapy in Young Adults with Hyperthyroidism of Graves' Disease.. By: Dunn, John T.. Annals of Internal Medicine, Jun84, Vol. 100 Issue 6, p891, 3p

30, 31 http://www.endocrineweb.com/conditions/thyroid-cancer/thyroid-cancer

32   Continuing Controversies in the Management of Thyroid Nodules. By: Castro, M. Regina; Gharib, Hossein. Annals of Internal Medicine, 6/7/2005, Vol. 142 Issue 11, p926-W-217, 7p

33   Radioiodine therapy (RAI) for Graves' disease (GD) and the effect on ophthalmopathy: a systematic review. By: Acharya, Shamasunder H.; Avenell, Alison; Philip, Sam; Burr, Jennifer; Bevan, John S.; Abraham, Prakash. Clinical Endocrinology, Dec2008, Vol. 69 Issue 6, p943-950, 8p, 4 Diagrams, 2 Charts

34   Brownstein, Dr. David. Iodine, Why You Need It, Why You Can't Live Without It. 2009: 91

35   Brownstein, Dr. David. Iodine, Why You Need It, Why You Can't Live Without It. 2009: 42-43

Index

168, 172, 179, 181, 182, 231
copper deficiency 98, 99, 223
copper toxicity 99, 223
corticosteroids 61, 163, 165, 167
cortisol levels 4, 45, 63, 64, 65, 71

D
dairy 78, 79, 84, 86, 111, 196
Danish population 106
dentistry model 192
DHEA 45, 65
Diagnos-Techs 63, 66, 85, 86, 92, 239
digestion 29, 76, 77
digestive enzymes 76, 79, 199
distilled water 90

E
Eleuthero 96, 101, 197
elimination diet 86
ELISA/EIA panel 85, 92
environmental toxins 11, 30, 31, 32, 55,
    57, 69, 109, 110, 113, 115, 116, 195
estrogen 85, 111, 112, 116, 225
estrogen dominance 225
exercise 67, 68, 78, 110, 176
exophthalmos 163, 164

F
fiber 77, 80, 241
Fine Needle Aspiration 158
food allergies 85, 86, 92, 199
food diary 92
Free T3 100
Free T4 18, 123, 132

G
gastrointestinal tract 85
genetics 12, 30, 32, 52, 117, 118, 119,
    121, 122
GI Health Panel 85, 92
Gliadin AB 65

glutathione 100
gluten 65, 78, 79, 83, 84, 86, 196, 197,
    217, 218
goiter 24, 218, 222, 224
goitrogens 90, 91, 92
Graves Disease 14, 24, 25, 124, 215,
    236, 237
Graves' ophthalmopathy 163, 168
Gymnema 73, 74

H
hair mineral analysis 45, 126, 221, 225,
    226
Hashimoto's Thyroiditis 2, 21, 51, 106,
    109, 111, 124, 125, 163, 203, 215,
    223, 236
heavy metals 226
herbs 11, 12, 37, 93, 94, 95, 98, 100,
    101, 150, 152, 155, 171, 172, 173,
    174, 175, 176, 180, 181, 182, 183,
    184, 185, 186, 187, 191, 192, 193,
    195, 201, 228
high cortisol 45, 64
high energy levels 71
homeopathy 228, 229
hyperthyroid diet 11, 84, 88, 92
hyperthyroidism 1, 2, 3, 4, 7, 8, 9, 10,
    11, 12, 13, 18, 20, 21, 22, 23, 24, 25,
    27, 28, 29, 30, 31, 32, 34, 42, 44, 45,
    46, 47, 48, 49, 52, 59, 61, 62, 68, 69,
    71, 72, 74, 85, 88, 90, 91, 92, 93, 94,
    95, 97, 98, 99, 100, 101, 103, 106,
    107, 117, 118, 126, 127, 129, 130,
    132, 133, 134, 135, 136, 144, 145,
    146, 147, 151, 152, 153, 154, 157,
    158, 161, 167, 169, 170, 171, 172,
    173, 174, 175, 177, 179, 180, 182,
    184, 185, 189, 191, 197, 202, 203,
    204, 205, 206, 207, 209, 211, 212,
    214, 215, 218, 219, 220, 221, 222,
    223, 224, 225, 227, 228, 229, 231,

FREE WEBINARS
On Natural Hyperthyroid Treatment Methods

IF YOU HAVE hyperthyroidism or Graves' Disease and want to do everything you can to avoid radioactive iodine treatment and thyroid surgery, then I highly recommend attending one of our free webinars on natural thyroid health (specifically the one called "Natural Treatment Solutions For Hyperthyroidism & Graves' Disease). The webinars are approximately 45 minutes long, and they provide plenty of valuable information for those people looking to restore their health by following a natural treatment protocol. For more information on how to register for an upcoming free webinar, visit www.GravesDiseaseBook.com and click on the "Free Webinars" link.

SPECIAL FREE GIFT FROM THE AUTHOR

As a way of thanking you for purchasing this book, I'd like to offer you a free audio CD** entitled "The 6 Steps On How To Treat Hyperthyroidism & Graves' Disease Through Natural Methods".

**There is a $2.95 fee for s/h ($6.95 for international orders)

Name: _____

Address: _____

City: _____ State: _____ Zip: _____

Phone: _____

Payment Options:

❏ Check: Make check or money in the amount of $2.95 to Natural Endocrine Solutions, and mail to the following address:

Natural Endocrine Solutions
4100 Carmel Road Ste B #106
Charlotte, NC 28226

❏ Credit Card: Type of card (circle one)
Visa   Mastercard   Discover   American Express
Credit Card #: _____ Exp Date: _____

Please Copy This Page And Fax to 1-888-380-1153
(or scan and email this form to info@GravesDiseaseBook.com)

CPSIA information can be obtained at www.ICGtesting.com
Printed in the USA
244989LV00004B/4/P